oxygen™
WOMEN'S FITNESS

NO
PAIN
NO
GAIN

TRAINING
JOURNAL

Published by Robert Kennedy Publishing
400 Matheson Blvd. West
Mississauga, ON
L5R 3M1 Canada
Visit us at **www.oxygenmag.com**

Managing Senior Production Editor: Wendy Morley
Online and Associate Editor: Vinita Persaud
Junior Production Editor: Cali Hoffman
Art Director: Gabriella Caruso Marques
Acting Art Director: Jessica Pensabene
Editorial Designer: Ellie Jeon

Cover Photography: Paul Buceta
Cover Model: Amber Elizabeth

Library and Archives Canada Cataloguing in Publication

No pain, no gain : training journal / [from the editors of Oxygen].

ISBN 978-1-55210-071-4

1. Weight training for women. 2. Exercise for women.

GV546.6.W64N6 2009   613.7'045   C2009-906094-9

10 9 8 7 6 5 4 3 2 1

Distributed in Canada by
NBN (National Book Network)
67 Mowat Avenue, Suite 241
Toronto, ON
M6K 3E3

Distributed in USA by
NBN (National Book Network)
15200 NBN Way
Blue Ridge Summit, PA
17214

Printed in Canada

IMPORTANT

The information in this book reflects the author's experiences and opinions and is not intended to replace medical advice.

Before beginning this or any nutritional or exercise regimen, consult your physician to be sure it is appropriate for you. Ask for a physical stress test.

GENERAL INFORMATION

NAME _____

ADDRESS _____

CITY _____ STATE _____ ZIP _____

PHONE _____

FAX _____

COMPANY NAME _____

ADDRESS _____

CITY _____ STATE _____ ZIP _____

PHONE _____

FAX _____

EMERGENCY INFORMATION

NOTIFY _____ RELATIONSHIP _____

PHONE _____ WORK PHONE _____

ADDRESS _____

CITY _____ STATE _____ ZIP _____

OR NOTIFY _____ RELATIONSHIP _____

PHONE _____ WORK PHONE _____

ADDRESS _____

CITY _____ STATE _____ ZIP _____

MEDICAL INFORMATION

PHYSICIAN _____ PHONE _____

INSURANCE/HMO _____

BLOOD TYPE _____ ALLERGIES _____

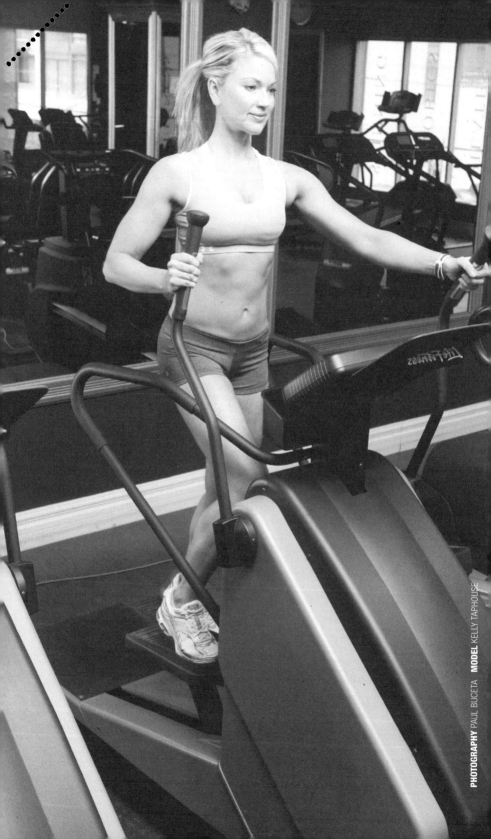

INTRODUCTION

Getting to the gym on a regular basis is an important part of my life. I've experienced firsthand the changes resistance training can have on the body – it has brought me to my best shape. Not only has this way of training helped me make constant improvements to my physique, it's the perfect outlet for shaking off the day's stress. A workout never fails to boost my mood and energize me along with making me stronger and healthier.

But in order to keep my gym workouts working for me, I have to go in with a plan. If I don't have my workout completely mapped out, I won't make the most of my time.

This is where *Oxygen's No Pain No Gain Training Journal* comes into play. If you incorporate it into your lifestyle, you will soon see improvements, guaranteed. By keeping a record of your exercises, sets, reps and weights every time you work out, you will see more definition, decrease your body fat and bust through plateaus.

This journal makes it simple to track and record your progress. Plus, it offers muscle group illustrations, motivating photos of your favorite fitness models and a calendar for monthly goals and reminders.

No Pain No Gain will become your best training partner to date. It's easy to use and compact (to fit perfectly in your gym bag). It will help keep you pumped and looking forward to each and every workout.

Stacy K

Stacy Kennedy, Editor-in-Chief
of *Oxygen* magazine

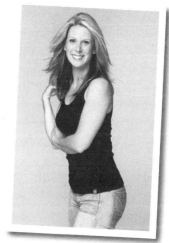

PHOTOGRAPHY PAUL BUCETA

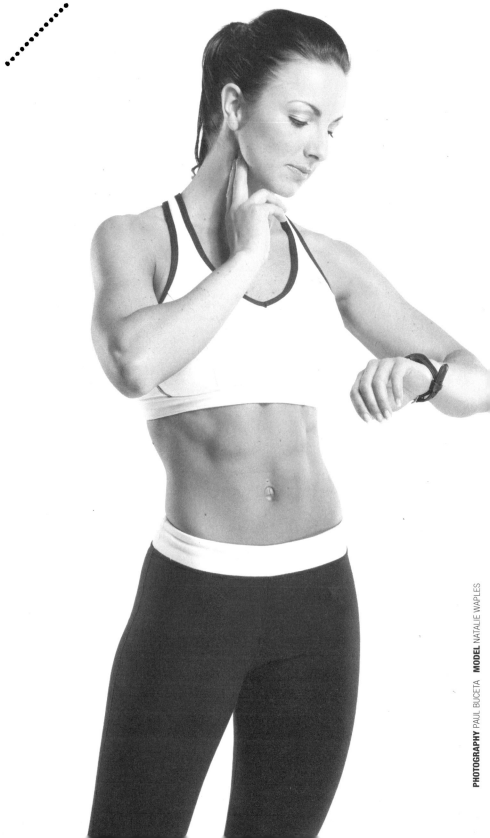

CALCULATING INTENSITY LEVELS

Your heart rate is a good indicator of your intensity level during your cardio workouts. If it is between 55 and 80 percent of your maximum heart rate, or MHR, then you are training aerobically. This means "with oxygen," and is an activity that can be carried out for long periods of time. If your heart rate is between 80 and 100 percent of your MHR, then you are training anaerobically. You will be able to train this way for short bursts, but not for extended periods.

Cardio training should be done for a minimum of 20 minutes at a time. You can go steadily and stay in a given heart-rate zone, or you can do interval training, in which case you work in both the aerobic and anaerobic zones. Interval training is by far the most effective for improving cardiovascular fitness and for burning calories, but this is an intensity technique and you'll have to work your way up to it! Be sure to visit your doctor for a stress test before beginning any exercise program.

To figure out your maximum heart rate, subtract your age from 220. Multiply by 0.55, 0.65, 0.75 and 0.85 to determine your optimal heart-rate training ranges.
- **BEGINNERS** should should stay between 55 and 65 percent of their MHR.
- **INTERMEDIATES** can work in the range of 65 to 75 percent.
- **ADVANCED** trainers can work steadily in the 75-to 85-percent range, and can go even higher for short bursts, if they're in good enough condition.

TARGET HEART-RATE ZONES
Beats Per Minute

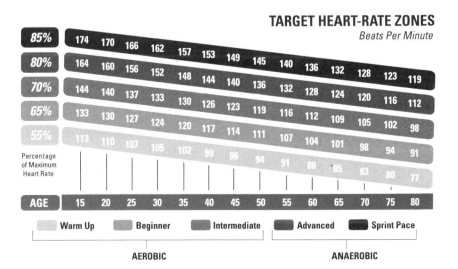

Percentage of Maximum Heart Rate	15	20	25	30	35	40	45	50	55	60	65	70	75	80
85%	174	170	166	162	157	153	149	145	140	136	132	128	123	119
80%	164	160	156	152	148	144	140	136	132	128	124	120	116	112
70%	144	140	137	133	130	126	123	119	116	112	109	105	102	98
65%	133	130	127	124	120	117	114	111	107	104	101	98	94	91
55%	113	110	107	105	102	99	96	94	91	88	85	83	80	77

AGE | 15 | 20 | 25 | 30 | 35 | 40 | 45 | 50 | 55 | 60 | 65 | 70 | 75 | 80

Warm Up   Beginner   Intermediate   Advanced   Sprint Pace

AEROBIC   ANAEROBIC

MUSCLE GROUPS

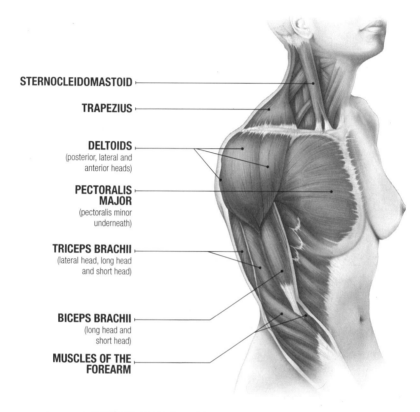

STERNOCLEIDOMASTOID

TRAPEZIUS

DELTOIDS
(posterior, lateral and
anterior heads)

**PECTORALIS
MAJOR**
(pectoralis minor
underneath)

TRICEPS BRACHII
(lateral head, long head
and short head)

BICEPS BRACHII
(long head and
short head)

**MUSCLES OF THE
FOREARM**

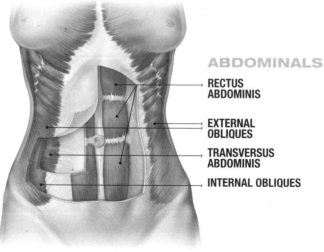

ABDOMINALS

**RECTUS
ABDOMINIS**

**EXTERNAL
OBLIQUES**

**TRANSVERSUS
ABDOMINIS**

INTERNAL OBLIQUES

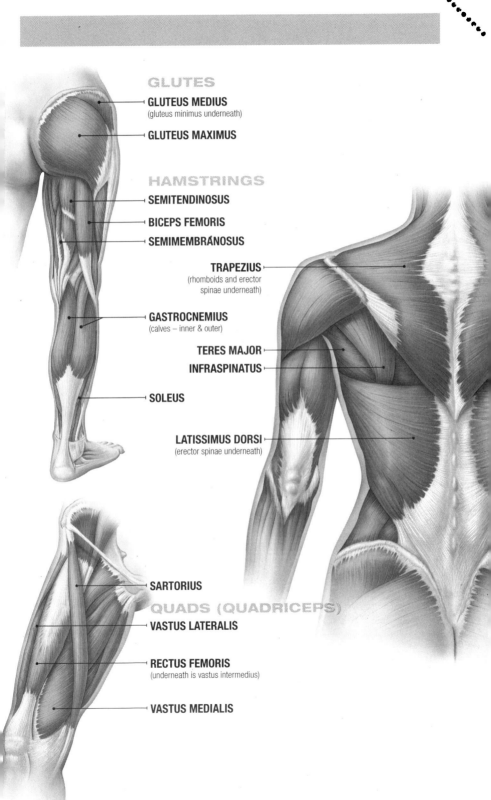

GLUTES

GLUTEUS MEDIUS
(gluteus minimus underneath)

GLUTEUS MAXIMUS

HAMSTRINGS

SEMITENDINOSUS

BICEPS FEMORIS

SEMIMEMBRÁNOSUS

TRAPEZIUS
(rhomboids and erector
spinae underneath)

GASTROCNEMIUS
(calves – inner & outer)

TERES MAJOR

INFRASPINATUS

SOLEUS

LATISSIMUS DORSI
(erector spinae underneath)

SARTORIUS

QUADS (QUADRICEPS)

VASTUS LATERALIS

RECTUS FEMORIS
(underneath is vastus intermedius)

VASTUS MEDIALIS

Record your weight and measurements on a monthly basis. This will help you to keep track of your progress throughout the year. You'll be surprised at how much progress you've made each month.

	DATE:	**DATE:**	**DATE:**
WEIGHT			
BODY-FAT PERCENTAGE			

MEASUREMENTS

	DATE:	DATE:	DATE:
CHEST			
WAIST			
HIP			
RIGHT THIGH			
LEFT THIGH			
RIGHT ARM - relaxed:			
- flexed:			
LEFT ARM - relaxed:			
- flexed:			
RIGHT CALF			
LEFT CALF			
FOREARM			

	DATE:	**DATE:**	**DATE:**
WEIGHT			
BODY-FAT PERCENTAGE			

MEASUREMENTS

CHEST			
WAIST			
HIP			
RIGHT THIGH			
LEFT THIGH			
RIGHT ARM - relaxed: - flexed:			
LEFT ARM - relaxed: - flexed:			
RIGHT CALF			
LEFT CALF			
FOREARM			

GOALS AND REMINDERS

Set your short-term and long-term goals and reassess yourself monthly as a reminder. Doing so will keep you motivated and on track. Give yourself reasonable goals to work toward. Rather than trying to lose 20 pounds in one week, strive for two pounds. You can try for 20 pounds over time.

JANUARY

WEEK 1: ☐

WEEK 2: ☐

WEEK 3: ☐

WEEK 4: ☐

WEEK 5 (IF NECESSARY): ☐

MONTHLY GOAL:

☐

FEBRUARY

WEEK 1: ☐

WEEK 2: ☐

WEEK 3: ☐

WEEK 4: ☐

WEEK 5 (IF NECESSARY): ☐

MONTHLY GOAL:

☐

MARCH

WEEK 1: ☐

WEEK 2: ☐

WEEK 3: ☐

WEEK 4: ☐

WEEK 5 (IF NECESSARY): ☐

MONTHLY GOAL:

☐

APRIL

WEEK 1: ☐

WEEK 2: ☐

WEEK 3: ☐

WEEK 4: ☐

WEEK 5 (IF NECESSARY): ☐

MONTHLY GOAL:

☐

MAY

WEEK 1: ☐

WEEK 2: ☐

WEEK 3: ☐

WEEK 4: ☐

WEEK 5 (IF NECESSARY): ☐

MONTHLY GOAL:

☐

JUNE

WEEK 1: ☐

WEEK 2: ☐

WEEK 3: ☐

WEEK 4: ☐

WEEK 5 (IF NECESSARY): ☐

MONTHLY GOAL:

☐

GOALS AND REMINDERS

Set your short-term and long-term goals and reassess yourself monthly as a reminder. Doing so will keep you motivated and on track. Give yourself reasonable goals to work toward. Rather than trying to lose 20 pounds in one week, strive for two pounds. You can try for 20 pounds over time.

JULY

WEEK 1: ☐

WEEK 2: ☐

WEEK 3: ☐

WEEK 4: ☐

WEEK 5 (IF NECESSARY): ☐

MONTHLY GOAL:

☐

AUGUST

WEEK 1: ☐

WEEK 2: ☐

WEEK 3: ☐

WEEK 4: ☐

WEEK 5 (IF NECESSARY): ☐

MONTHLY GOAL:

☐

SEPTEMBER

WEEK 1: ☐

WEEK 2: ☐

WEEK 3: ☐

WEEK 4: ☐

WEEK 5 (IF NECESSARY): ☐

MONTHLY GOAL:

☐

OCTOBER

WEEK 1: ☐

WEEK 2: ☐

WEEK 3: ☐

WEEK 4: ☐

WEEK 5 (IF NECESSARY): ☐

MONTHLY GOAL:

☐

WEEK 1: ☐

WEEK 2: ☐

WEEK 3: ☐

WEEK 4: ☐

WEEK 5 (IF NECESSARY): ☐

MONTHLY GOAL:

☐

DECEMBER

WEEK 1: ☐

WEEK 2: ☐

WEEK 3: ☐

WEEK 4: ☐

WEEK 5 (IF NECESSARY): ☐

MONTHLY GOAL:

☐

TODAY'S TRAINING

DATE

EXERCISE	SET 1	SET 2	SET 3	SET 4	SET 5	SET 6	SET 7	SET 8
	WEIGHT	WEIGHT	WEIGHT	WEIGHT	WEIGHT	WEIGHT	WEIGHT	WEIGHT
	REPS	REPS	REPS	REPS	REPS	REPS	REPS	REPS

CARDIO/NOTES:

TODAY'S TRAINING

DATE

EXERCISE	SET 1 WEIGHT REPS	SET 2 WEIGHT REPS	SET 3 WEIGHT REPS	SET 4 WEIGHT REPS	SET 5 WEIGHT REPS	SET 6 WEIGHT REPS	SET 7 WEIGHT REPS	SET 8 WEIGHT REPS

CARDIO/NOTES:

TODAY'S TRAINING

EXERCISE	SET 1 WEIGHT / REPS	SET 2 WEIGHT / REPS	SET 3 WEIGHT / REPS	SET 4 WEIGHT / REPS	SET 5 WEIGHT / REPS	SET 6 WEIGHT / REPS	SET 7 WEIGHT / REPS	SET 8 WEIGHT / REPS

CARDIO/NOTES:

" Conditions are never just right. People who delay action until all factors are favorable do nothing. "

– William Feather

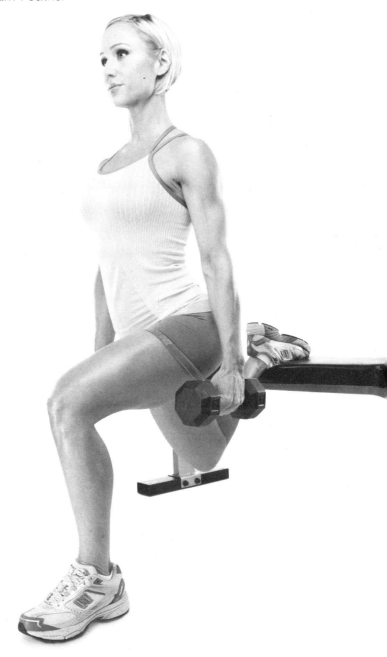

PHOTOGRAPHY PAUL BUCETA **MODEL** JAMIE EASON

TODAY'S TRAINING

EXERCISE	SET 1		SET 2		SET 3		SET 4		SET 5		SET 6		SET 7		SET 8	
	WEIGHT		WEIGHT		WEIGHT		WEIGHT		WEIGHT		WEIGHT		WEIGHT		WEIGHT	
	REPS		REPS		REPS		REPS		REPS		REPS		REPS		REPS	

CARDIO/NOTES:

TODAY'S TRAINING

DATE

EXERCISE	SET 1 WEIGHT REPS	SET 2 WEIGHT REPS	SET 3 WEIGHT REPS	SET 4 WEIGHT REPS	SET 5 WEIGHT REPS	SET 6 WEIGHT REPS	SET 7 WEIGHT REPS	SET 8 WEIGHT REPS

CARDIO/NOTES:

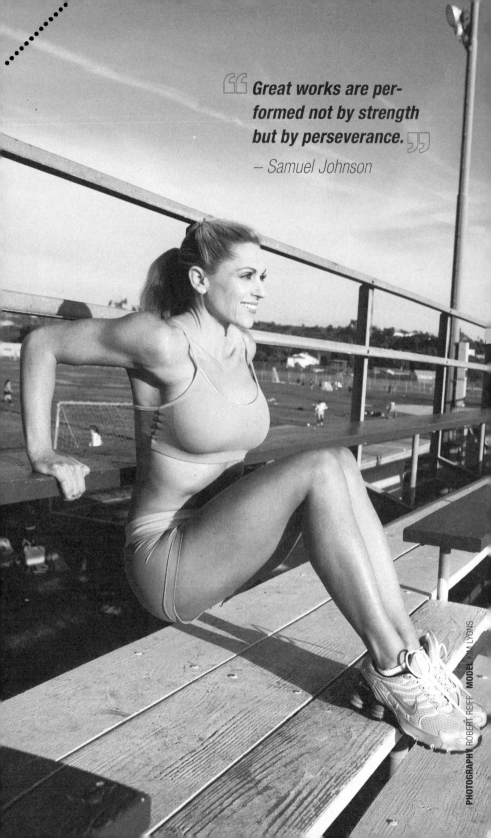

> **Great works are performed not by strength but by perseverance.**
> – *Samuel Johnson*

TODAY'S TRAINING

DATE

EXERCISE	SET 1 WEIGHT REPS	SET 2 WEIGHT REPS	SET 3 WEIGHT REPS	SET 4 WEIGHT REPS	SET 5 WEIGHT REPS	SET 6 WEIGHT REPS	SET 7 WEIGHT REPS	SET 8 WEIGHT REPS

CARDIO/NOTES:

TODAY'S TRAINING

DATE

EXERCISE	SET 1 WEIGHT	SET 2 WEIGHT	SET 3 WEIGHT	SET 4 WEIGHT	SET 5 WEIGHT	SET 6 WEIGHT	SET 7 WEIGHT	SET 8 WEIGHT
	REPS	REPS	REPS	REPS	REPS	REPS	REPS	REPS

CARDIO/NOTES:

TODAY'S TRAINING

DATE

EXERCISE	SET 1 WEIGHT REPS	SET 2 WEIGHT REPS	SET 3 WEIGHT REPS	SET 4 WEIGHT REPS	SET 5 WEIGHT REPS	SET 6 WEIGHT REPS	SET 7 WEIGHT REPS	SET 8 WEIGHT REPS

CARDIO/NOTES:

TODAY'S TRAINING

DATE

EXERCISE	SET 1	SET 2	SET 3	SET 4	SET 5	SET 6	SET 7	SET 8
	WEIGHT	WEIGHT	WEIGHT	WEIGHT	WEIGHT	WEIGHT	WEIGHT	WEIGHT
	REPS	REPS	REPS	REPS	REPS	REPS	REPS	REPS

CARDIO/NOTES:

If you doubt you can accomplish something, then you can't accomplish it. You have to have confidence in your ability, and then be tough enough to follow through.

– Rosalynn Smith Carter

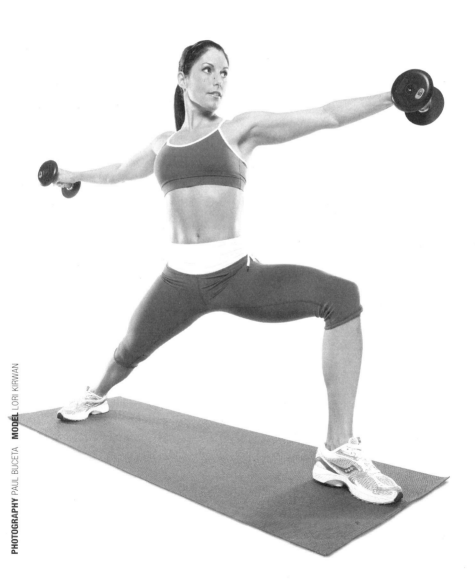

TODAY'S TRAINING

DATE

EXERCISE	SET 1	SET 2	SET 3	SET 4	SET 5	SET 6	SET 7	SET 8
	WEIGHT	WEIGHT	WEIGHT	WEIGHT	WEIGHT	WEIGHT	WEIGHT	WEIGHT
	REPS	REPS	REPS	REPS	REPS	REPS	REPS	REPS

CARDIO/NOTES:

TODAY'S TRAINING

EXERCISE	SET 1 WEIGHT	SET 2 WEIGHT	SET 3 WEIGHT	SET 4 WEIGHT	SET 5 WEIGHT	SET 6 WEIGHT	SET 7 WEIGHT	SET 8 WEIGHT
	REPS	REPS	REPS	REPS	REPS	REPS	REPS	REPS

CARDIO/NOTES:

TODAY'S TRAINING

DATE

EXERCISE	SET 1 WEIGHT REPS	SET 2 WEIGHT REPS	SET 3 WEIGHT REPS	SET 4 WEIGHT REPS	SET 5 WEIGHT REPS	SET 6 WEIGHT REPS	SET 7 WEIGHT REPS	SET 8 WEIGHT REPS

CARDIO/NOTES:

TODAY'S TRAINING

DATE

EXERCISE	SET 1 WEIGHT REPS	SET 2 WEIGHT REPS	SET 3 WEIGHT REPS	SET 4 WEIGHT REPS	SET 5 WEIGHT REPS	SET 6 WEIGHT REPS	SET 7 WEIGHT REPS	SET 8 WEIGHT REPS

CARDIO/NOTES:

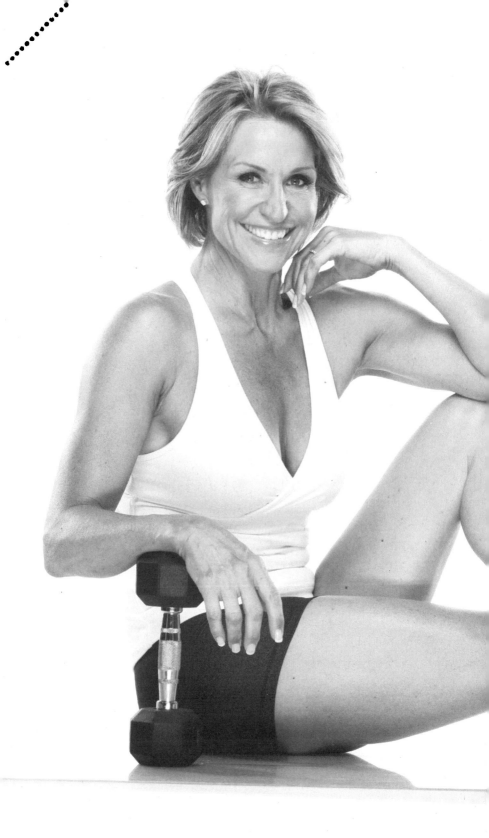

" *There are three types of people in this world: those who make things happen, those who watch things happen and those who wonder what happened. We all have a choice. You can decide which type of person you want to be. I have always chosen to be in the first group.* **"**

— Mary Kay Ash

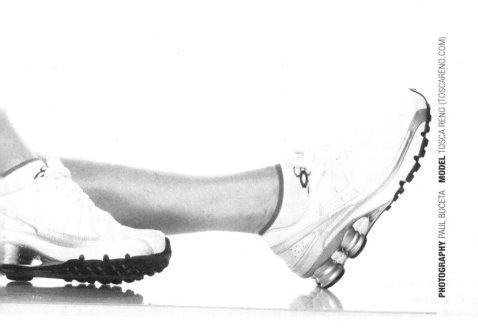

TODAY'S TRAINING

DATE

EXERCISE	SET 1 WEIGHT REPS	SET 2 WEIGHT REPS	SET 3 WEIGHT REPS	SET 4 WEIGHT REPS	SET 5 WEIGHT REPS	SET 6 WEIGHT REPS	SET 7 WEIGHT REPS	SET 8 WEIGHT REPS

CARDIO/NOTES:

TODAY'S TRAINING

DATE

EXERCISE	SET 1 WEIGHT	SET 2 WEIGHT	SET 3 WEIGHT	SET 4 WEIGHT	SET 5 WEIGHT	SET 6 WEIGHT	SET 7 WEIGHT	SET 8 WEIGHT
	REPS	REPS	REPS	REPS	REPS	REPS	REPS	REPS

CARDIO/NOTES:

TODAY'S TRAINING

DATE

EXERCISE	SET 1 WEIGHT	SET 2 WEIGHT	SET 3 WEIGHT	SET 4 WEIGHT	SET 5 WEIGHT	SET 6 WEIGHT	SET 7 WEIGHT	SET 8 WEIGHT
	REPS	REPS	REPS	REPS	REPS	REPS	REPS	REPS

CARDIO/NOTES:

TODAY'S TRAINING

DATE

EXERCISE	SET 1 WEIGHT / REPS	SET 2 WEIGHT / REPS	SET 3 WEIGHT / REPS	SET 4 WEIGHT / REPS	SET 5 WEIGHT / REPS	SET 6 WEIGHT / REPS	SET 7 WEIGHT / REPS	SET 8 WEIGHT / REPS

CARDIO/NOTES:

TODAY'S TRAINING

DATE

EXERCISE	SET 1 WEIGHT REPS	SET 2 WEIGHT REPS	SET 3 WEIGHT REPS	SET 4 WEIGHT REPS	SET 5 WEIGHT REPS	SET 6 WEIGHT REPS	SET 7 WEIGHT REPS	SET 8 WEIGHT REPS

CARDIO/NOTES:

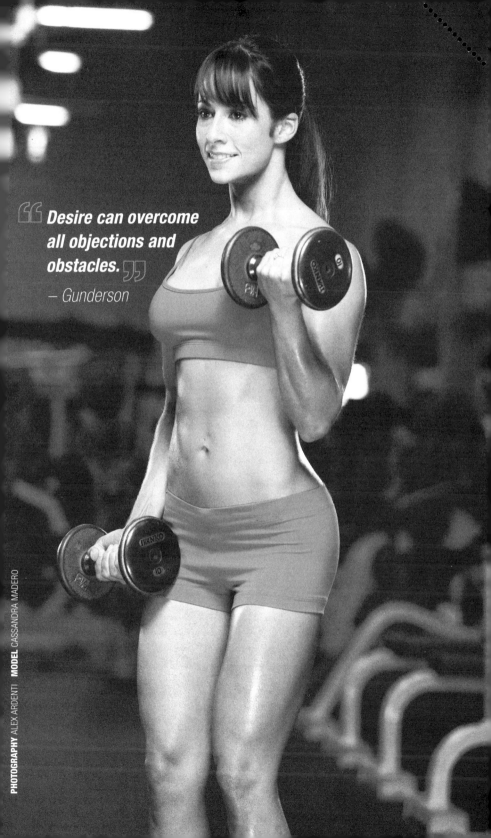

> **Desire can overcome all objections and obstacles.**
> — *Gunderson*

TODAY'S TRAINING

DATE

EXERCISE	SET 1	SET 2	SET 3	SET 4	SET 5	SET 6	SET 7	SET 8
	WEIGHT	WEIGHT	WEIGHT	WEIGHT	WEIGHT	WEIGHT	WEIGHT	WEIGHT
	REPS	REPS	REPS	REPS	REPS	REPS	REPS	REPS

CARDIO/NOTES:

TODAY'S TRAINING

DATE

EXERCISE	SET 1 WEIGHT	SET 2 WEIGHT	SET 3 WEIGHT	SET 4 WEIGHT	SET 5 WEIGHT	SET 6 WEIGHT	SET 7 WEIGHT	SET 8 WEIGHT
	REPS	REPS	REPS	REPS	REPS	REPS	REPS	REPS

CARDIO/NOTES:

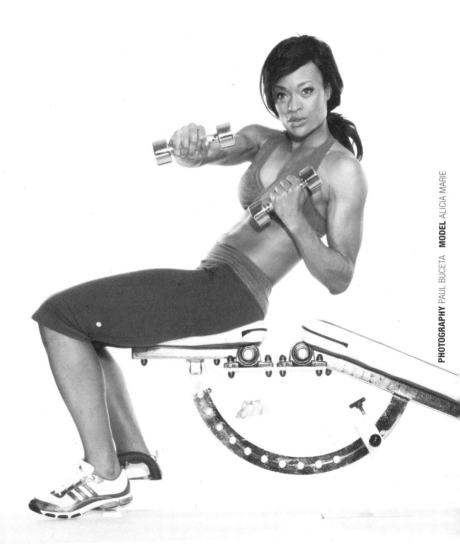

Crystallize your goals. Make a plan for achieving them and set yourself a deadline. Then, with supreme confidence, determination and disregard for obstacles and other people's criticism, carry out your plan.

– Paul J. Meyer

TODAY'S TRAINING

DATE

EXERCISE	SET 1 WEIGHT REPS	SET 2 WEIGHT REPS	SET 3 WEIGHT REPS	SET 4 WEIGHT REPS	SET 5 WEIGHT REPS	SET 6 WEIGHT REPS	SET 7 WEIGHT REPS	SET 8 WEIGHT REPS

CARDIO/NOTES:

TODAY'S TRAINING

EXERCISE	SET 1		SET 2		SET 3		SET 4		SET 5		SET 6		SET 7		SET 8	
	WEIGHT	REPS	WEIGHT	REPS	WEIGHT	REPS	WEIGHT	REPS	WEIGHT	REPS	WEIGHT	REPS	WEIGHT	REPS	WEIGHT	REPS

CARDIO/NOTES:

TODAY'S TRAINING

DATE

EXERCISE	SET 1		SET 2		SET 3		SET 4		SET 5		SET 6		SET 7		SET 8	
	WEIGHT	REPS	WEIGHT	REPS	WEIGHT	REPS	WEIGHT	REPS	WEIGHT	REPS	WEIGHT	REPS	WEIGHT	REPS	WEIGHT	REPS

CARDIO/NOTES:

TODAY'S TRAINING

DATE

EXERCISE	SET 1 WEIGHT REPS	SET 2 WEIGHT REPS	SET 3 WEIGHT REPS	SET 4 WEIGHT REPS	SET 5 WEIGHT REPS	SET 6 WEIGHT REPS	SET 7 WEIGHT REPS	SET 8 WEIGHT REPS

CARDIO/NOTES:

TODAY'S TRAINING

DATE

EXERCISE	SET 1 WEIGHT / REPS	SET 2 WEIGHT / REPS	SET 3 WEIGHT / REPS	SET 4 WEIGHT / REPS	SET 5 WEIGHT / REPS	SET 6 WEIGHT / REPS	SET 7 WEIGHT / REPS	SET 8 WEIGHT / REPS

CARDIO/NOTES:

TODAY'S TRAINING

DATE

EXERCISE	SET 1 WEIGHT REPS	SET 2 WEIGHT REPS	SET 3 WEIGHT REPS	SET 4 WEIGHT REPS	SET 5 WEIGHT REPS	SET 6 WEIGHT REPS	SET 7 WEIGHT REPS	SET 8 WEIGHT REPS

CARDIO/NOTES:

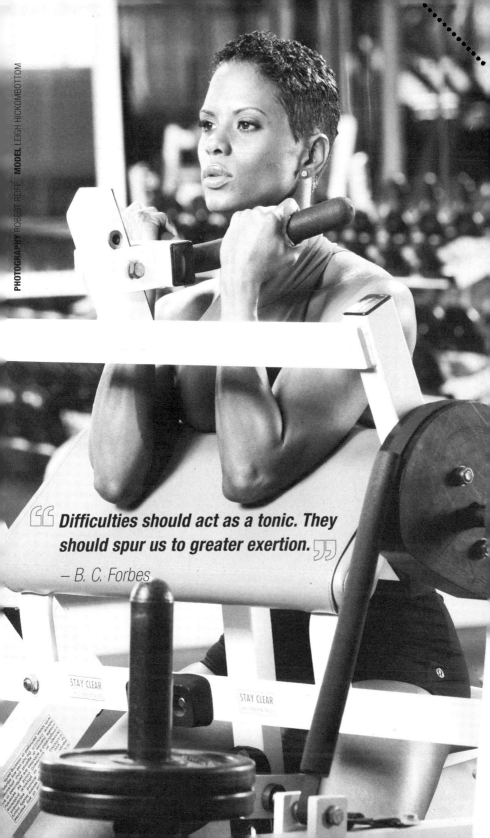

Difficulties should act as a tonic. They should spur us to greater exertion.

– B. C. Forbes

STAY CLEAR

STAY CLEAR

TODAY'S TRAINING

DATE

EXERCISE	SET 1 WEIGHT	SET 2 WEIGHT	SET 3 WEIGHT	SET 4 WEIGHT	SET 5 WEIGHT	SET 6 WEIGHT	SET 7 WEIGHT	SET 8 WEIGHT
	REPS	REPS	REPS	REPS	REPS	REPS	REPS	REPS

CARDIO/NOTES:

TODAY'S TRAINING

DATE

EXERCISE	SET 1 WEIGHT	SET 1 REPS	SET 2 WEIGHT	SET 2 REPS	SET 3 WEIGHT	SET 3 REPS	SET 4 WEIGHT	SET 4 REPS	SET 5 WEIGHT	SET 5 REPS	SET 6 WEIGHT	SET 6 REPS	SET 7 WEIGHT	SET 7 REPS	SET 8 WEIGHT	SET 8 REPS

CARDIO/NOTES:

TODAY'S TRAINING

DATE

EXERCISE	SET 1 WEIGHT	SET 2 WEIGHT	SET 3 WEIGHT	SET 4 WEIGHT	SET 5 WEIGHT	SET 6 WEIGHT	SET 7 WEIGHT	SET 8 WEIGHT
	REPS	REPS	REPS	REPS	REPS	REPS	REPS	REPS

CARDIO/NOTES:

TODAY'S TRAINING

DATE

EXERCISE	SET 1 WEIGHT	SET 2 WEIGHT	SET 3 WEIGHT	SET 4 WEIGHT	SET 5 WEIGHT	SET 6 WEIGHT	SET 7 WEIGHT	SET 8 WEIGHT
	REPS	REPS	REPS	REPS	REPS	REPS	REPS	REPS

CARDIO/NOTES:

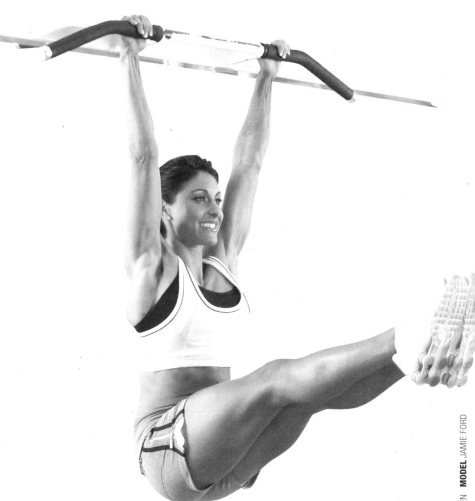

Great things are not done by impulse, but by a series of small things brought together.

– Vincent Van Gogh

PHOTOGRAPHY CORY SORENSEN   MODEL JAMIE FORD

TODAY'S TRAINING

DATE

EXERCISE	SET 1	SET 2	SET 3	SET 4	SET 5	SET 6	SET 7	SET 8
	WEIGHT	WEIGHT	WEIGHT	WEIGHT	WEIGHT	WEIGHT	WEIGHT	WEIGHT
	REPS	REPS	REPS	REPS	REPS	REPS	REPS	REPS

CARDIO/NOTES:

TODAY'S TRAINING

EXERCISE	SET 1		SET 2		SET 3		SET 4		SET 5		SET 6		SET 7		SET 8	
	WEIGHT	REPS	WEIGHT	REPS	WEIGHT	REPS	WEIGHT	REPS	WEIGHT	REPS	WEIGHT	REPS	WEIGHT	REPS	WEIGHT	REPS

CARDIO/NOTES:

TODAY'S TRAINING

DATE

EXERCISE	SET 1 WEIGHT REPS	SET 2 WEIGHT REPS	SET 3 WEIGHT REPS	SET 4 WEIGHT REPS	SET 5 WEIGHT REPS	SET 6 WEIGHT REPS	SET 7 WEIGHT REPS	SET 8 WEIGHT REPS

CARDIO/NOTES:

TODAY'S TRAINING

DATE

EXERCISE	SET 1 WEIGHT / REPS	SET 2 WEIGHT / REPS	SET 3 WEIGHT / REPS	SET 4 WEIGHT / REPS	SET 5 WEIGHT / REPS	SET 6 WEIGHT / REPS	SET 7 WEIGHT / REPS	SET 8 WEIGHT / REPS

CARDIO/NOTES:

TODAY'S TRAINING

DATE

EXERCISE	SET 1	SET 2	SET 3	SET 4	SET 5	SET 6	SET 7	SET 8
	WEIGHT	WEIGHT	WEIGHT	WEIGHT	WEIGHT	WEIGHT	WEIGHT	WEIGHT
	REPS	REPS	REPS	REPS	REPS	REPS	REPS	REPS

CARDIO/NOTES:

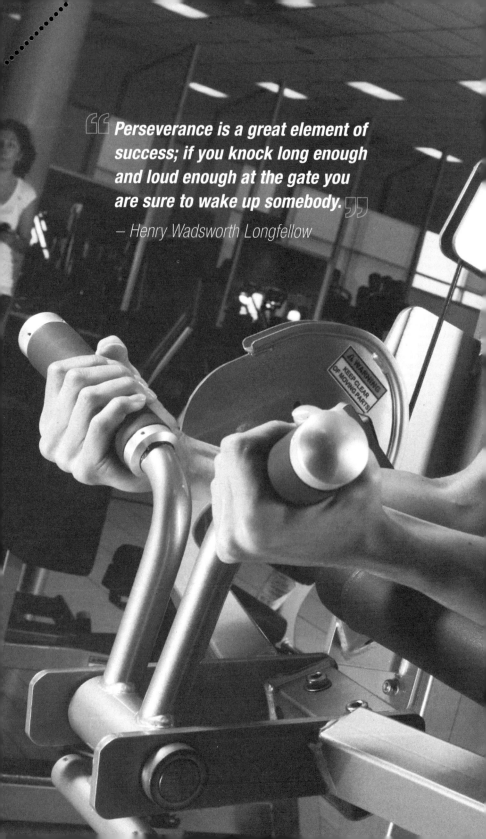

Perseverance is a great element of success; if you knock long enough and loud enough at the gate you are sure to wake up somebody.

— Henry Wadsworth Longfellow

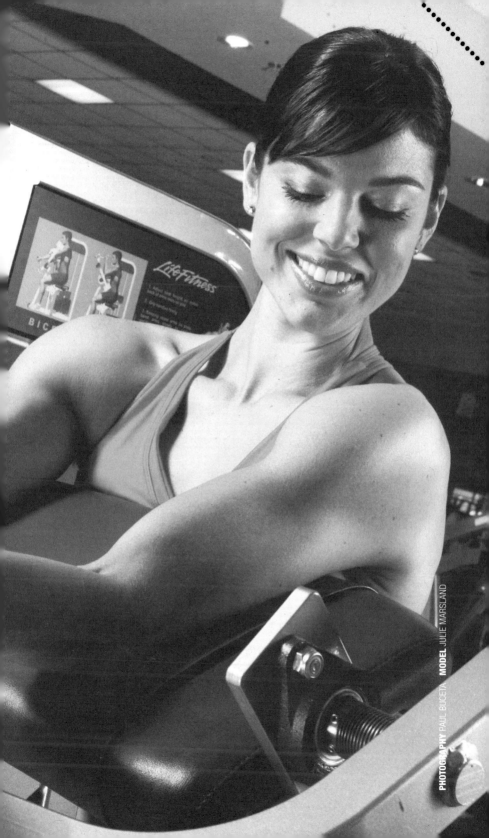

TODAY'S TRAINING

DATE

EXERCISE	SET 1 WEIGHT	SET 2 WEIGHT	SET 3 WEIGHT	SET 4 WEIGHT	SET 5 WEIGHT	SET 6 WEIGHT	SET 7 WEIGHT	SET 8 WEIGHT
	REPS	REPS	REPS	REPS	REPS	REPS	REPS	REPS

CARDIO/NOTES:

TODAY'S TRAINING

DATE

EXERCISE	SET 1	SET 2	SET 3	SET 4	SET 5	SET 6	SET 7	SET 8
	WEIGHT	WEIGHT	WEIGHT	WEIGHT	WEIGHT	WEIGHT	WEIGHT	WEIGHT
	REPS	REPS	REPS	REPS	REPS	REPS	REPS	REPS

CARDIO/NOTES:

TODAY'S TRAINING

DATE

EXERCISE	SET 1 WEIGHT REPS	SET 2 WEIGHT REPS	SET 3 WEIGHT REPS	SET 4 WEIGHT REPS	SET 5 WEIGHT REPS	SET 6 WEIGHT REPS	SET 7 WEIGHT REPS	SET 8 WEIGHT REPS

CARDIO/NOTES:

TODAY'S TRAINING

DATE

EXERCISE	SET 1	SET 2	SET 3	SET 4	SET 5	SET 6	SET 7	SET 8
	WEIGHT	WEIGHT	WEIGHT	WEIGHT	WEIGHT	WEIGHT	WEIGHT	WEIGHT
	REPS	REPS	REPS	REPS	REPS	REPS	REPS	REPS

CARDIO/NOTES:

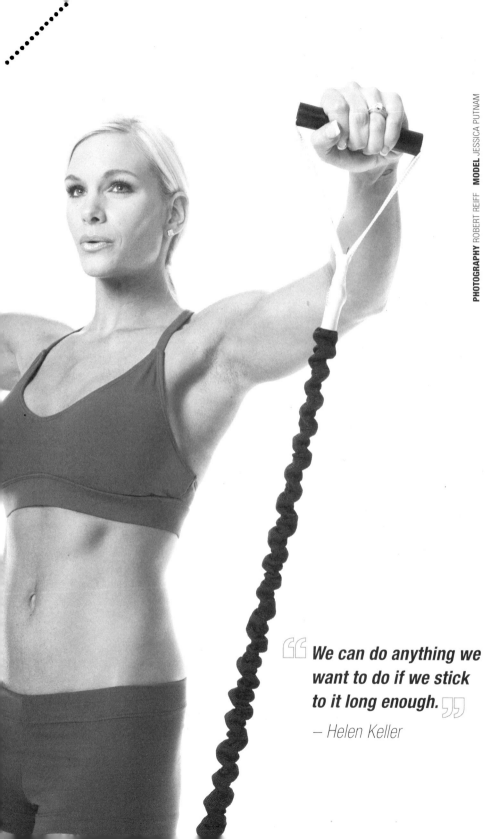

We can do anything we want to do if we stick to it long enough.

— *Helen Keller*

TODAY'S TRAINING

DATE

EXERCISE	SET 1	SET 2	SET 3	SET 4	SET 5	SET 6	SET 7	SET 8
	WEIGHT	WEIGHT	WEIGHT	WEIGHT	WEIGHT	WEIGHT	WEIGHT	WEIGHT
	REPS	REPS	REPS	REPS	REPS	REPS	REPS	REPS

CARDIO/NOTES:

TODAY'S TRAINING

DATE

EXERCISE	SET 1 WEIGHT	SET 2 WEIGHT	SET 3 WEIGHT	SET 4 WEIGHT	SET 5 WEIGHT	SET 6 WEIGHT	SET 7 WEIGHT	SET 8 WEIGHT
	REPS	REPS	REPS	REPS	REPS	REPS	REPS	REPS

CARDIO/NOTES:

TODAY'S TRAINING

DATE

EXERCISE	SET 1 WEIGHT REPS	SET 2 WEIGHT REPS	SET 3 WEIGHT REPS	SET 4 WEIGHT REPS	SET 5 WEIGHT REPS	SET 6 WEIGHT REPS	SET 7 WEIGHT REPS	SET 8 WEIGHT REPS

CARDIO/NOTES:

TODAY'S TRAINING

EXERCISE	SET 1	SET 2	SET 3	SET 4	SET 5	SET 6	SET 7	SET 8
	WEIGHT	WEIGHT	WEIGHT	WEIGHT	WEIGHT	WEIGHT	WEIGHT	WEIGHT
	REPS	REPS	REPS	REPS	REPS	REPS	REPS	REPS

CARDIO/NOTES:

TODAY'S TRAINING

EXERCISE	SET 1	SET 2	SET 3	SET 4	SET 5	SET 6	SET 7	SET 8
	WEIGHT	WEIGHT	WEIGHT	WEIGHT	WEIGHT	WEIGHT	WEIGHT	WEIGHT
	REPS	REPS	REPS	REPS	REPS	REPS	REPS	REPS

CARDIO/NOTES:

TODAY'S TRAINING

EXERCISE	SET 1		SET 2		SET 3		SET 4		SET 5		SET 6		SET 7		SET 8	
	WEIGHT	REPS	WEIGHT	REPS	WEIGHT	REPS	WEIGHT	REPS	WEIGHT	REPS	WEIGHT	REPS	WEIGHT	REPS	WEIGHT	REPS

CARDIO/NOTES:

TODAY'S TRAINING

DATE

EXERCISE	SET 1 WEIGHT / REPS	SET 2 WEIGHT / REPS	SET 3 WEIGHT / REPS	SET 4 WEIGHT / REPS	SET 5 WEIGHT / REPS	SET 6 WEIGHT / REPS	SET 7 WEIGHT / REPS	SET 8 WEIGHT / REPS

CARDIO/NOTES:

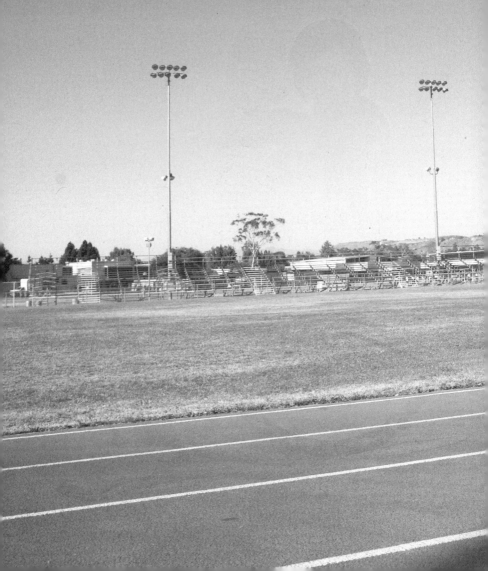

> **Within each of us is a hidden store of determination. Determination to keep us in the race when all seems lost.**
>
> – Roger Dawson

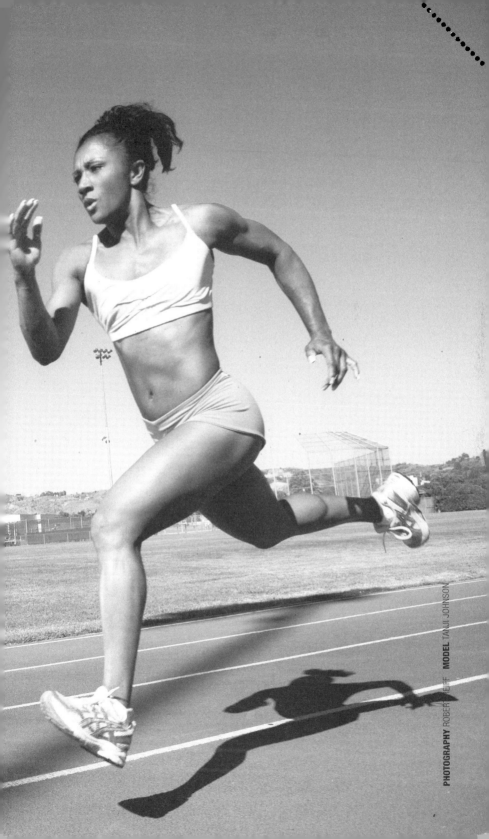

TODAY'S TRAINING

DATE

EXERCISE	SET 1 WEIGHT REPS	SET 2 WEIGHT REPS	SET 3 WEIGHT REPS	SET 4 WEIGHT REPS	SET 5 WEIGHT REPS	SET 6 WEIGHT REPS	SET 7 WEIGHT REPS	SET 8 WEIGHT REPS

CARDIO/NOTES:

TODAY'S TRAINING

DATE

EXERCISE	SET 1 WEIGHT	SET 2 WEIGHT	SET 3 WEIGHT	SET 4 WEIGHT	SET 5 WEIGHT	SET 6 WEIGHT	SET 7 WEIGHT	SET 8 WEIGHT
	REPS	REPS	REPS	REPS	REPS	REPS	REPS	REPS

CARDIO/NOTES:

TODAY'S TRAINING

DATE

EXERCISE	SET 1 WEIGHT	SET 2 WEIGHT	SET 3 WEIGHT	SET 4 WEIGHT	SET 5 WEIGHT	SET 6 WEIGHT	SET 7 WEIGHT	SET 8 WEIGHT
	REPS	REPS	REPS	REPS	REPS	REPS	REPS	REPS

CARDIO/NOTES:

TODAY'S TRAINING

DATE

EXERCISE	SET 1 WEIGHT REPS	SET 2 WEIGHT REPS	SET 3 WEIGHT REPS	SET 4 WEIGHT REPS	SET 5 WEIGHT REPS	SET 6 WEIGHT REPS	SET 7 WEIGHT REPS	SET 8 WEIGHT REPS

CARDIO/NOTES:

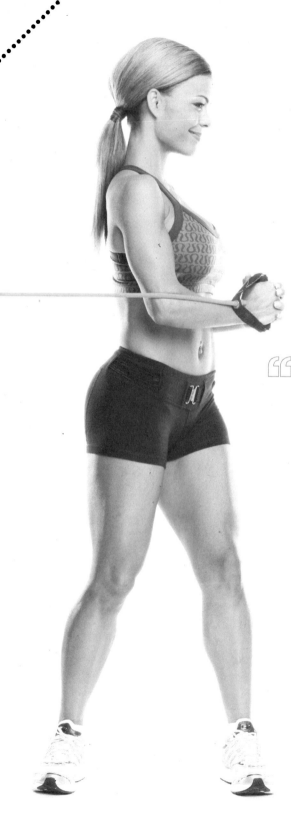

> **Determination gives you the resolve to keep going in spite of the roadblocks that lay before you.**
> – Denis Waitley

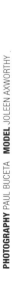

TODAY'S TRAINING

DATE

EXERCISE	SET 1	SET 2	SET 3	SET 4	SET 5	SET 6	SET 7	SET 8
	WEIGHT	WEIGHT	WEIGHT	WEIGHT	WEIGHT	WEIGHT	WEIGHT	WEIGHT
	REPS	REPS	REPS	REPS	REPS	REPS	REPS	REPS

CARDIO/NOTES:

TODAY'S TRAINING

DATE

EXERCISE	SET 1 WEIGHT REPS	SET 2 WEIGHT REPS	SET 3 WEIGHT REPS	SET 4 WEIGHT REPS	SET 5 WEIGHT REPS	SET 6 WEIGHT REPS	SET 7 WEIGHT REPS	SET 8 WEIGHT REPS

CARDIO/NOTES:

TODAY'S TRAINING

DATE

EXERCISE	SET 1 WEIGHT	SET 2 WEIGHT	SET 3 WEIGHT	SET 4 WEIGHT	SET 5 WEIGHT	SET 6 WEIGHT	SET 7 WEIGHT	SET 8 WEIGHT
	REPS	REPS	REPS	REPS	REPS	REPS	REPS	REPS

CARDIO/NOTES:

TODAY'S TRAINING

DATE

EXERCISE	SET 1	SET 2	SET 3	SET 4	SET 5	SET 6	SET 7	SET 8
	WEIGHT	WEIGHT	WEIGHT	WEIGHT	WEIGHT	WEIGHT	WEIGHT	WEIGHT
	REPS	REPS	REPS	REPS	REPS	REPS	REPS	REPS

CARDIO/NOTES:

TODAY'S TRAINING

DATE

EXERCISE	SET 1 WEIGHT	SET 2 WEIGHT	SET 3 WEIGHT	SET 4 WEIGHT	SET 5 WEIGHT	SET 6 WEIGHT	SET 7 WEIGHT	SET 8 WEIGHT
	REPS	REPS	REPS	REPS	REPS	REPS	REPS	REPS

CARDIO/NOTES:

TODAY'S TRAINING

DATE

EXERCISE	SET 1 WEIGHT	SET 2 WEIGHT	SET 3 WEIGHT	SET 4 WEIGHT	SET 5 WEIGHT	SET 6 WEIGHT	SET 7 WEIGHT	SET 8 WEIGHT
	REPS	REPS	REPS	REPS	REPS	REPS	REPS	REPS

CARDIO/NOTES:

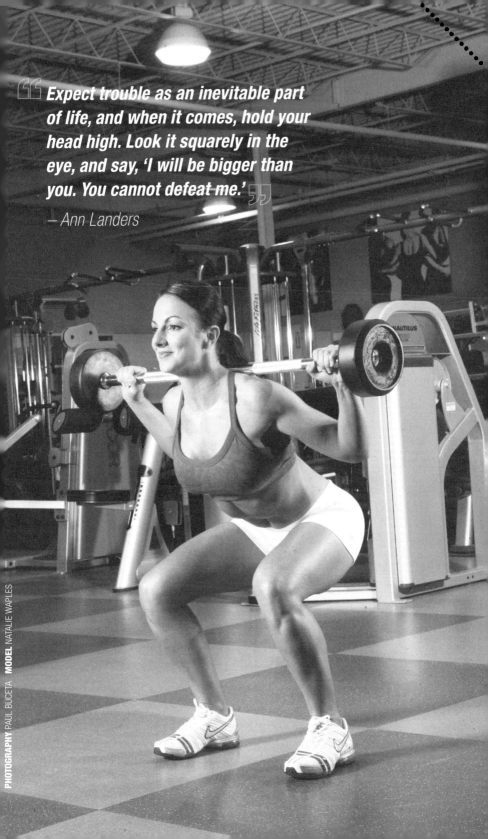

> **Expect trouble as an inevitable part of life, and when it comes, hold your head high. Look it squarely in the eye, and say, 'I will be bigger than you. You cannot defeat me.'**
>
> *— Ann Landers*

TODAY'S TRAINING

DATE

EXERCISE	SET 1 WEIGHT / REPS	SET 2 WEIGHT / REPS	SET 3 WEIGHT / REPS	SET 4 WEIGHT / REPS	SET 5 WEIGHT / REPS	SET 6 WEIGHT / REPS	SET 7 WEIGHT / REPS	SET 8 WEIGHT / REPS

CARDIO/NOTES:

TODAY'S TRAINING

DATE

EXERCISE	SET 1 WEIGHT	SET 2 WEIGHT	SET 3 WEIGHT	SET 4 WEIGHT	SET 5 WEIGHT	SET 6 WEIGHT	SET 7 WEIGHT	SET 8 WEIGHT
	REPS	REPS	REPS	REPS	REPS	REPS	REPS	REPS

CARDIO/NOTES:

TODAY'S TRAINING

DATE

EXERCISE	SET 1	SET 2	SET 3	SET 4	SET 5	SET 6	SET 7	SET 8
	WEIGHT	WEIGHT	WEIGHT	WEIGHT	WEIGHT	WEIGHT	WEIGHT	WEIGHT
	REPS	REPS	REPS	REPS	REPS	REPS	REPS	REPS

CARDIO/NOTES:

TODAY'S TRAINING

DATE

EXERCISE	SET 1 WEIGHT	SET 2 WEIGHT	SET 3 WEIGHT	SET 4 WEIGHT	SET 5 WEIGHT	SET 6 WEIGHT	SET 7 WEIGHT	SET 8 WEIGHT
	REPS	REPS	REPS	REPS	REPS	REPS	REPS	REPS

CARDIO/NOTES:

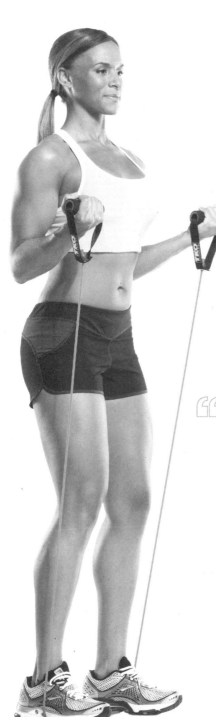

PHOTOGRAPHY PAUL BUCETA **MODEL** JASMINE CORBETT

The most important step in any major accomplishment is setting a specific goal. This enables you to keep your mind focused on your goal and off the many obstacles that will arise when you're striving to do your best.

— *Kurt Thomas*

TODAY'S TRAINING

DATE

EXERCISE	SET 1		SET 2		SET 3		SET 4		SET 5		SET 6		SET 7		SET 8	
	WEIGHT	REPS	WEIGHT	REPS	WEIGHT	REPS	WEIGHT	REPS	WEIGHT	REPS	WEIGHT	REPS	WEIGHT	REPS	WEIGHT	REPS

CARDIO/NOTES:

TODAY'S TRAINING

DATE

EXERCISE	SET 1 WEIGHT REPS	SET 2 WEIGHT REPS	SET 3 WEIGHT REPS	SET 4 WEIGHT REPS	SET 5 WEIGHT REPS	SET 6 WEIGHT REPS	SET 7 WEIGHT REPS	SET 8 WEIGHT REPS

CARDIO/NOTES:

TODAY'S TRAINING

DATE

EXERCISE	SET 1		SET 2		SET 3		SET 4		SET 5		SET 6		SET 7		SET 8	
	WEIGHT	REPS	WEIGHT	REPS	WEIGHT	REPS	WEIGHT	REPS	WEIGHT	REPS	WEIGHT	REPS	WEIGHT	REPS	WEIGHT	REPS

CARDIO/NOTES:

TODAY'S TRAINING

DATE

EXERCISE	SET 1	SET 2	SET 3	SET 4	SET 5	SET 6	SET 7	SET 8
	WEIGHT	WEIGHT	WEIGHT	WEIGHT	WEIGHT	WEIGHT	WEIGHT	WEIGHT
	REPS	REPS	REPS	REPS	REPS	REPS	REPS	REPS

CARDIO/NOTES:

TODAY'S TRAINING

DATE

EXERCISE	SET 1	SET 2	SET 3	SET 4	SET 5	SET 6	SET 7	SET 8
	WEIGHT	WEIGHT	WEIGHT	WEIGHT	WEIGHT	WEIGHT	WEIGHT	WEIGHT
	REPS	REPS	REPS	REPS	REPS	REPS	REPS	REPS

CARDIO/NOTES:

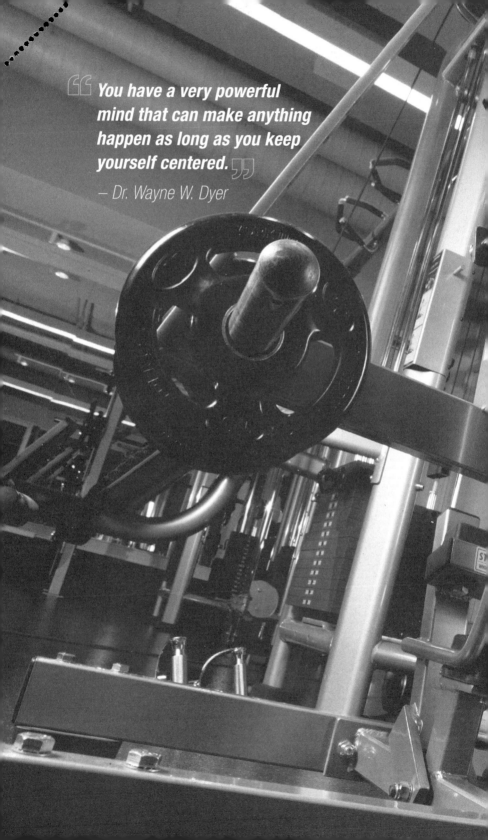

> "You have a very powerful mind that can make anything happen as long as you keep yourself centered."
> — Dr. Wayne W. Dyer

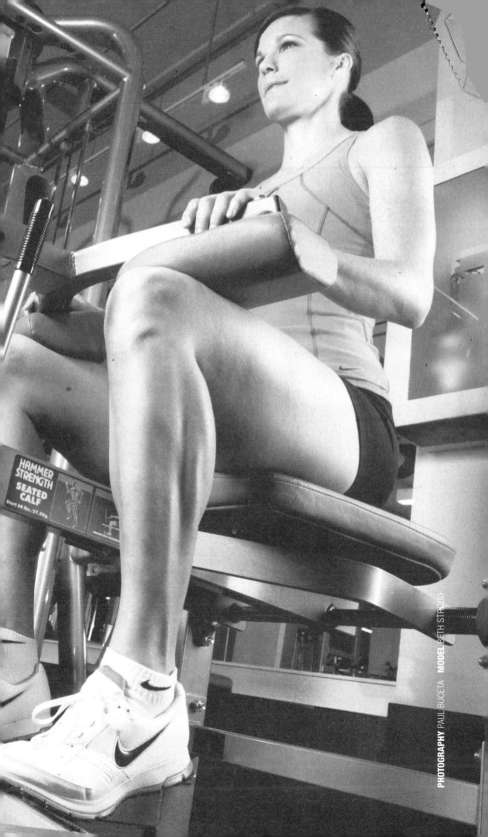

HAMMER
STRENGTH
SEATED
CALF
Start 60 lbs. / 27.2Kg.

TODAY'S TRAINING

DATE

EXERCISE	SET 1 WEIGHT REPS	SET 2 WEIGHT REPS	SET 3 WEIGHT REPS	SET 4 WEIGHT REPS	SET 5 WEIGHT REPS	SET 6 WEIGHT REPS	SET 7 WEIGHT REPS	SET 8 WEIGHT REPS

CARDIO/NOTES:

TODAY'S TRAINING

DATE

EXERCISE	SET 1 WEIGHT / REPS	SET 2 WEIGHT / REPS	SET 3 WEIGHT / REPS	SET 4 WEIGHT / REPS	SET 5 WEIGHT / REPS	SET 6 WEIGHT / REPS	SET 7 WEIGHT / REPS	SET 8 WEIGHT / REPS

CARDIO/NOTES:

TODAY'S TRAINING

DATE

EXERCISE	SET 1 WEIGHT REPS	SET 2 WEIGHT REPS	SET 3 WEIGHT REPS	SET 4 WEIGHT REPS	SET 5 WEIGHT REPS	SET 6 WEIGHT REPS	SET 7 WEIGHT REPS	SET 8 WEIGHT REPS

CARDIO/NOTES:

TODAY'S TRAINING

DATE

EXERCISE	SET 1		SET 2		SET 3		SET 4		SET 5		SET 6		SET 7		SET 8	
	WEIGHT		WEIGHT		WEIGHT		WEIGHT		WEIGHT		WEIGHT		WEIGHT		WEIGHT	
	REPS		REPS		REPS		REPS		REPS		REPS		REPS		REPS	

CARDIO/NOTES:

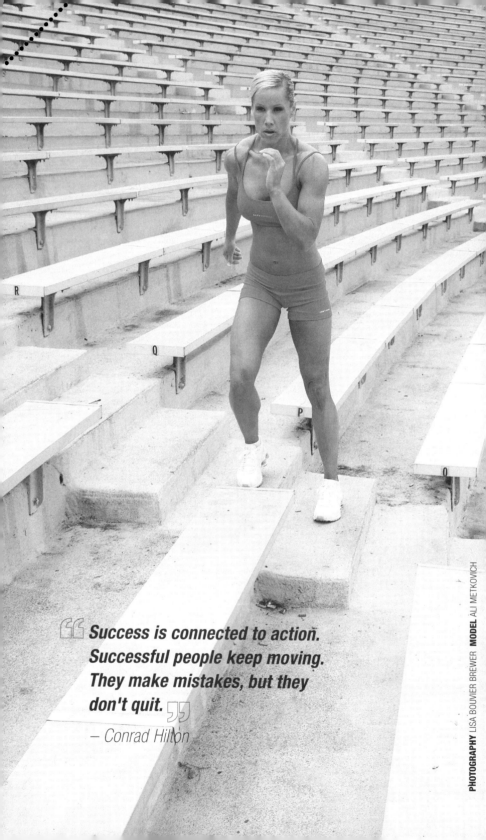

> **Success is connected to action. Successful people keep moving. They make mistakes, but they don't quit.**
>
> – Conrad Hilton

PHOTOGRAPHY LISA BOUVIER BREWER **MODEL** ALI METKOVICH

TODAY'S TRAINING

EXERCISE	SET 1	SET 2	SET 3	SET 4	SET 5	SET 6	SET 7	SET 8
	WEIGHT	WEIGHT	WEIGHT	WEIGHT	WEIGHT	WEIGHT	WEIGHT	WEIGHT
	REPS	REPS	REPS	REPS	REPS	REPS	REPS	REPS

CARDIO/NOTES:

TODAY'S TRAINING

DATE

EXERCISE	SET 1 WEIGHT REPS	SET 2 WEIGHT REPS	SET 3 WEIGHT REPS	SET 4 WEIGHT REPS	SET 5 WEIGHT REPS	SET 6 WEIGHT REPS	SET 7 WEIGHT REPS	SET 8 WEIGHT REPS

CARDIO/NOTES:

TODAY'S TRAINING

DATE

EXERCISE	SET 1		SET 2		SET 3		SET 4		SET 5		SET 6		SET 7		SET 8	
	WEIGHT	REPS	WEIGHT	REPS	WEIGHT	REPS	WEIGHT	REPS	WEIGHT	REPS	WEIGHT	REPS	WEIGHT	REPS	WEIGHT	REPS

CARDIO/NOTES:

TODAY'S TRAINING

DATE

EXERCISE	SET 1 WEIGHT REPS	SET 2 WEIGHT REPS	SET 3 WEIGHT REPS	SET 4 WEIGHT REPS	SET 5 WEIGHT REPS	SET 6 WEIGHT REPS	SET 7 WEIGHT REPS	SET 8 WEIGHT REPS

CARDIO/NOTES:

TODAY'S TRAINING

DATE

EXERCISE	SET 1		SET 2		SET 3		SET 4		SET 5		SET 6		SET 7		SET 8	
	WEIGHT	REPS	WEIGHT	REPS	WEIGHT	REPS	WEIGHT	REPS	WEIGHT	REPS	WEIGHT	REPS	WEIGHT	REPS	WEIGHT	REPS

CARDIO/NOTES:

TODAY'S TRAINING

DATE

EXERCISE	SET 1 WEIGHT	SET 2 WEIGHT	SET 3 WEIGHT	SET 4 WEIGHT	SET 5 WEIGHT	SET 6 WEIGHT	SET 7 WEIGHT	SET 8 WEIGHT
	REPS	REPS	REPS	REPS	REPS	REPS	REPS	REPS

CARDIO/NOTES:

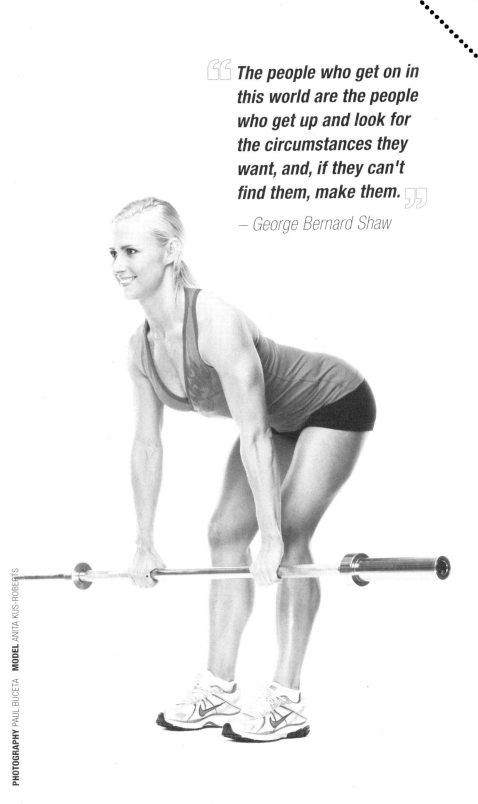

" The people who get on in this world are the people who get up and look for the circumstances they want, and, if they can't find them, make them. "

– *George Bernard Shaw*

TODAY'S TRAINING

DATE

EXERCISE	SET 1	SET 2	SET 3	SET 4	SET 5	SET 6	SET 7	SET 8
	WEIGHT	WEIGHT	WEIGHT	WEIGHT	WEIGHT	WEIGHT	WEIGHT	WEIGHT
	REPS	REPS	REPS	REPS	REPS	REPS	REPS	REPS

CARDIO/NOTES:

TODAY'S TRAINING

DATE

EXERCISE	SET 1	SET 2	SET 3	SET 4	SET 5	SET 6	SET 7	SET 8
	WEIGHT	WEIGHT	WEIGHT	WEIGHT	WEIGHT	WEIGHT	WEIGHT	WEIGHT
	REPS	REPS	REPS	REPS	REPS	REPS	REPS	REPS

CARDIO/NOTES:

TODAY'S TRAINING

EXERCISE	SET 1 WEIGHT REPS	SET 2 WEIGHT REPS	SET 3 WEIGHT REPS	SET 4 WEIGHT REPS	SET 5 WEIGHT REPS	SET 6 WEIGHT REPS	SET 7 WEIGHT REPS	SET 8 WEIGHT REPS

CARDIO/NOTES:

TODAY'S TRAINING

DATE

EXERCISE	SET 1		SET 2		SET 3		SET 4		SET 5		SET 6		SET 7		SET 8	
	WEIGHT	REPS	WEIGHT	REPS	WEIGHT	REPS	WEIGHT	REPS	WEIGHT	REPS	WEIGHT	REPS	WEIGHT	REPS	WEIGHT	REPS

CARDIO/NOTES:

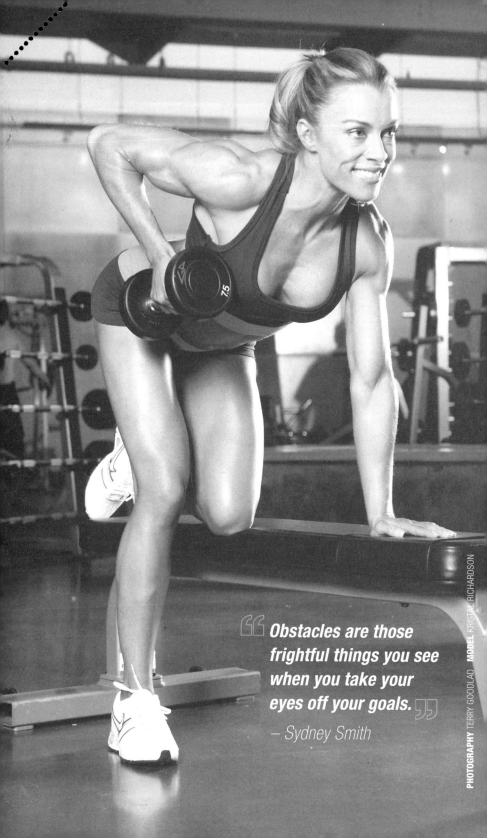

> **Obstacles are those frightful things you see when you take your eyes off your goals.**
> — *Sydney Smith*

TODAY'S TRAINING

DATE

EXERCISE	SET 1	SET 2	SET 3	SET 4	SET 5	SET 6	SET 7	SET 8
	WEIGHT	WEIGHT	WEIGHT	WEIGHT	WEIGHT	WEIGHT	WEIGHT	WEIGHT
	REPS	REPS	REPS	REPS	REPS	REPS	REPS	REPS

CARDIO/NOTES:

TODAY'S TRAINING

DATE

EXERCISE	SET 1 WEIGHT	SET 2 WEIGHT	SET 3 WEIGHT	SET 4 WEIGHT	SET 5 WEIGHT	SET 6 WEIGHT	SET 7 WEIGHT	SET 8 WEIGHT
	REPS	REPS	REPS	REPS	REPS	REPS	REPS	REPS

CARDIO/NOTES:

TODAY'S TRAINING

DATE

EXERCISE	SET 1	SET 2	SET 3	SET 4	SET 5	SET 6	SET 7	SET 8
	WEIGHT	WEIGHT	WEIGHT	WEIGHT	WEIGHT	WEIGHT	WEIGHT	WEIGHT
	REPS	REPS	REPS	REPS	REPS	REPS	REPS	REPS

CARDIO/NOTES:

TODAY'S TRAINING

EXERCISE	SET 1 WEIGHT REPS	SET 2 WEIGHT REPS	SET 3 WEIGHT REPS	SET 4 WEIGHT REPS	SET 5 WEIGHT REPS	SET 6 WEIGHT REPS	SET 7 WEIGHT REPS	SET 8 WEIGHT REPS

CARDIO/NOTES:

TODAY'S TRAINING

DATE

EXERCISE	SET 1	SET 2	SET 3	SET 4	SET 5	SET 6	SET 7	SET 8
	WEIGHT	WEIGHT	WEIGHT	WEIGHT	WEIGHT	WEIGHT	WEIGHT	WEIGHT
	REPS	REPS	REPS	REPS	REPS	REPS	REPS	REPS

CARDIO/NOTES:

TODAY'S TRAINING

DATE

EXERCISE	SET 1 WEIGHT	SET 2 WEIGHT	SET 3 WEIGHT	SET 4 WEIGHT	SET 5 WEIGHT	SET 6 WEIGHT	SET 7 WEIGHT	SET 8 WEIGHT
	REPS	REPS	REPS	REPS	REPS	REPS	REPS	REPS

CARDIO/NOTES:

TODAY'S TRAINING

DATE

EXERCISE	SET 1	SET 2	SET 3	SET 4	SET 5	SET 6	SET 7	SET 8
	WEIGHT	WEIGHT	WEIGHT	WEIGHT	WEIGHT	WEIGHT	WEIGHT	WEIGHT
	REPS	REPS	REPS	REPS	REPS	REPS	REPS	REPS

CARDIO/NOTES:

> **There is no chance, no destiny, no fate that can hinder or control the firm resolve of a determined soul.**
>
> — *Ella Wheeler Wilcox*

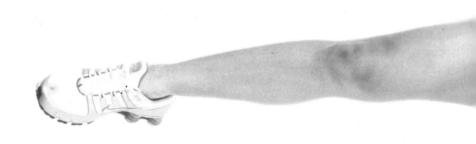

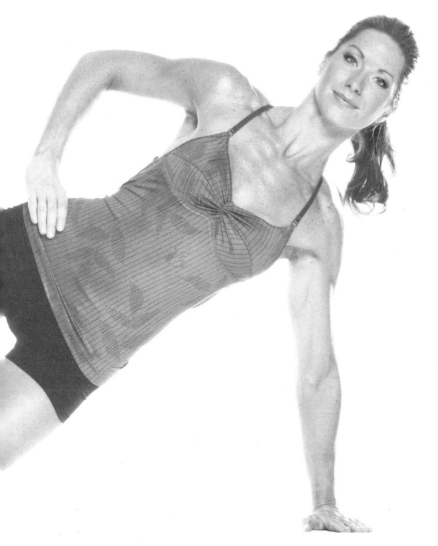

TODAY'S TRAINING

DATE

EXERCISE	SET 1	SET 2	SET 3	SET 4	SET 5	SET 6	SET 7	SET 8
	WEIGHT	WEIGHT	WEIGHT	WEIGHT	WEIGHT	WEIGHT	WEIGHT	WEIGHT
	REPS	REPS	REPS	REPS	REPS	REPS	REPS	REPS

CARDIO/NOTES:

TODAY'S TRAINING

DATE

EXERCISE	SET 1	SET 2	SET 3	SET 4	SET 5	SET 6	SET 7	SET 8
	WEIGHT	WEIGHT	WEIGHT	WEIGHT	WEIGHT	WEIGHT	WEIGHT	WEIGHT
	REPS	REPS	REPS	REPS	REPS	REPS	REPS	REPS

CARDIO/NOTES:

TODAY'S TRAINING

DATE

EXERCISE	SET 1 WEIGHT REPS	SET 2 WEIGHT REPS	SET 3 WEIGHT REPS	SET 4 WEIGHT REPS	SET 5 WEIGHT REPS	SET 6 WEIGHT REPS	SET 7 WEIGHT REPS	SET 8 WEIGHT REPS

CARDIO/NOTES:

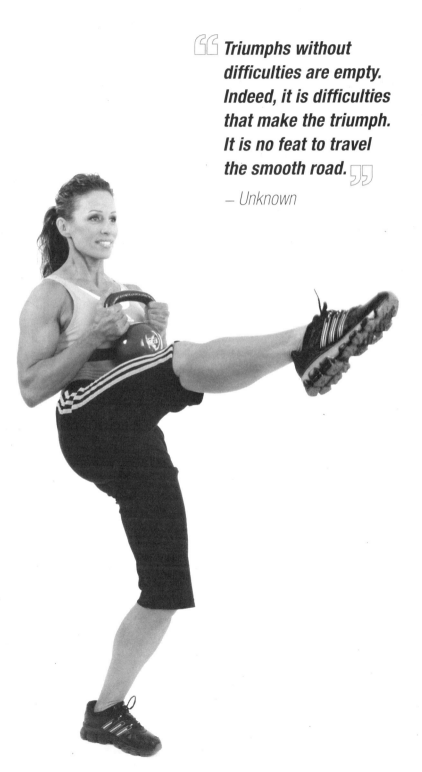

Triumphs without difficulties are empty. Indeed, it is difficulties that make the triumph. It is no feat to travel the smooth road.

— Unknown

TODAY'S TRAINING

DATE

EXERCISE	SET 1 WEIGHT REPS	SET 2 WEIGHT REPS	SET 3 WEIGHT REPS	SET 4 WEIGHT REPS	SET 5 WEIGHT REPS	SET 6 WEIGHT REPS	SET 7 WEIGHT REPS	SET 8 WEIGHT REPS

CARDIO/NOTES:

TODAY'S TRAINING

DATE

EXERCISE	SET 1	SET 2	SET 3	SET 4	SET 5	SET 6	SET 7	SET 8
	WEIGHT	WEIGHT	WEIGHT	WEIGHT	WEIGHT	WEIGHT	WEIGHT	WEIGHT
	REPS	REPS	REPS	REPS	REPS	REPS	REPS	REPS

CARDIO/NOTES:

TODAY'S TRAINING

DATE

EXERCISE	SET 1 WEIGHT / REPS	SET 2 WEIGHT / REPS	SET 3 WEIGHT / REPS	SET 4 WEIGHT / REPS	SET 5 WEIGHT / REPS	SET 6 WEIGHT / REPS	SET 7 WEIGHT / REPS	SET 8 WEIGHT / REPS

CARDIO/NOTES:

TODAY'S TRAINING

DATE

EXERCISE	SET 1 WEIGHT REPS	SET 2 WEIGHT REPS	SET 3 WEIGHT REPS	SET 4 WEIGHT REPS	SET 5 WEIGHT REPS	SET 6 WEIGHT REPS	SET 7 WEIGHT REPS	SET 8 WEIGHT REPS

CARDIO/NOTES:

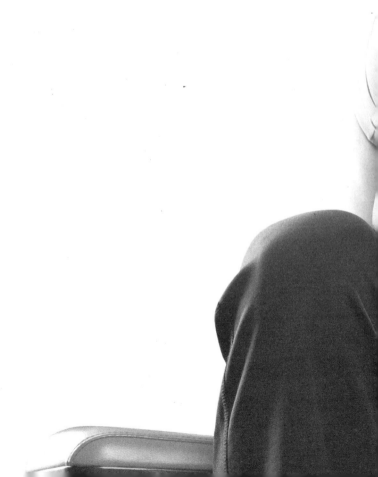

> **When we are motivated by goals that have deep meaning, by dreams that need completion, by pure love that needs expressing, then we truly live life.**
>
> – *Greg Anderson*

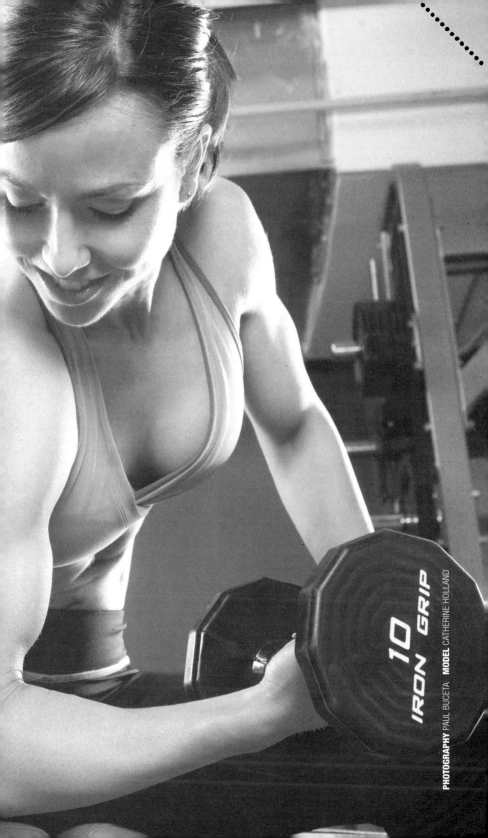

PHOTOGRAPHY PAUL BUCETA **MODEL** CATHERINE HOLLAND

10
IRON GRIP

TODAY'S TRAINING

EXERCISE	SET 1	SET 2	SET 3	SET 4	SET 5	SET 6	SET 7	SET 8
	WEIGHT	WEIGHT	WEIGHT	WEIGHT	WEIGHT	WEIGHT	WEIGHT	WEIGHT
	REPS	REPS	REPS	REPS	REPS	REPS	REPS	REPS

CARDIO/NOTES:

TODAY'S TRAINING

DATE

EXERCISE	SET 1		SET 2		SET 3		SET 4		SET 5		SET 6		SET 7		SET 8	
	WEIGHT	REPS	WEIGHT	REPS	WEIGHT	REPS	WEIGHT	REPS	WEIGHT	REPS	WEIGHT	REPS	WEIGHT	REPS	WEIGHT	REPS

CARDIO/NOTES:

EXERCISE	SET 1	SET 2	SET 3	SET 4	SET 5	SET 6	SET 7	SET 8
	WEIGHT	WEIGHT	WEIGHT	WEIGHT	WEIGHT	WEIGHT	WEIGHT	WEIGHT
	REPS	REPS	REPS	REPS	REPS	REPS	REPS	REPS

CARDIO/NOTES:

TODAY'S TRAINING

EXERCISE	SET 1 WEIGHT	SET 2 WEIGHT	SET 3 WEIGHT	SET 4 WEIGHT	SET 5 WEIGHT	SET 6 WEIGHT	SET 7 WEIGHT	SET 8 WEIGHT
	REPS	REPS	REPS	REPS	REPS	REPS	REPS	REPS

CARDIO/NOTES:

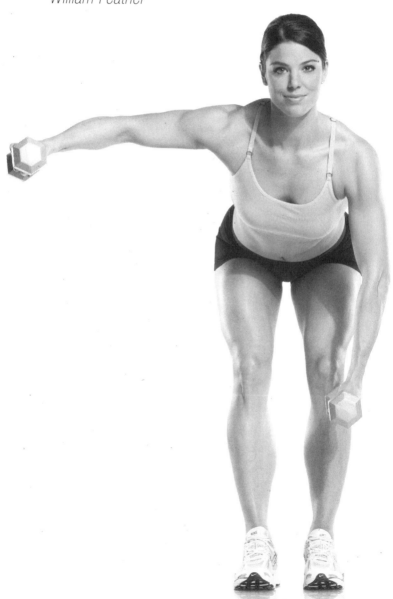

Success seems to be largely a matter of hanging on after others have let go.

– William Feather

TODAY'S TRAINING

DATE

EXERCISE	SET 1 WEIGHT / REPS	SET 2 WEIGHT / REPS	SET 3 WEIGHT / REPS	SET 4 WEIGHT / REPS	SET 5 WEIGHT / REPS	SET 6 WEIGHT / REPS	SET 7 WEIGHT / REPS	SET 8 WEIGHT / REPS

CARDIO/NOTES:

TODAY'S TRAINING

DATE

EXERCISE	SET 1 WEIGHT REPS	SET 2 WEIGHT REPS	SET 3 WEIGHT REPS	SET 4 WEIGHT REPS	SET 5 WEIGHT REPS	SET 6 WEIGHT REPS	SET 7 WEIGHT REPS	SET 8 WEIGHT REPS

CARDIO/NOTES:

TODAY'S TRAINING

DATE

EXERCISE	SET 1 WEIGHT	SET 2 WEIGHT	SET 3 WEIGHT	SET 4 WEIGHT	SET 5 WEIGHT	SET 6 WEIGHT	SET 7 WEIGHT	SET 8 WEIGHT
	REPS	REPS	REPS	REPS	REPS	REPS	REPS	REPS

CARDIO/NOTES:

TODAY'S TRAINING

DATE

EXERCISE	SET 1 WEIGHT	SET 2 WEIGHT	SET 3 WEIGHT	SET 4 WEIGHT	SET 5 WEIGHT	SET 6 WEIGHT	SET 7 WEIGHT	SET 8 WEIGHT
	REPS	REPS	REPS	REPS	REPS	REPS	REPS	REPS

CARDIO/NOTES:

TODAY'S TRAINING

DATE

EXERCISE	SET 1	SET 2	SET 3	SET 4	SET 5	SET 6	SET 7	SET 8
	WEIGHT	WEIGHT	WEIGHT	WEIGHT	WEIGHT	WEIGHT	WEIGHT	WEIGHT
	REPS	REPS	REPS	REPS	REPS	REPS	REPS	REPS

CARDIO/NOTES:

TODAY'S TRAINING

DATE

EXERCISE	SET 1		SET 2		SET 3		SET 4		SET 5		SET 6		SET 7		SET 8	
	WEIGHT	REPS	WEIGHT	REPS	WEIGHT	REPS	WEIGHT	REPS	WEIGHT	REPS	WEIGHT	REPS	WEIGHT	REPS	WEIGHT	REPS

CARDIO/NOTES:

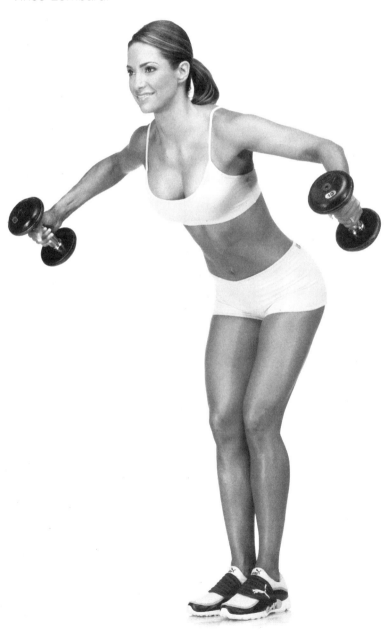

It's not whether you get knocked down. It's whether you get up again.

– Vince Lombardi

TODAY'S TRAINING

DATE

EXERCISE	SET 1 WEIGHT / REPS	SET 2 WEIGHT / REPS	SET 3 WEIGHT / REPS	SET 4 WEIGHT / REPS	SET 5 WEIGHT / REPS	SET 6 WEIGHT / REPS	SET 7 WEIGHT / REPS	SET 8 WEIGHT / REPS

CARDIO/NOTES:

TODAY'S TRAINING

DATE

EXERCISE	SET 1 WEIGHT	SET 2 WEIGHT	SET 3 WEIGHT	SET 4 WEIGHT	SET 5 WEIGHT	SET 6 WEIGHT	SET 7 WEIGHT	SET 8 WEIGHT
	REPS	REPS	REPS	REPS	REPS	REPS	REPS	REPS

CARDIO/NOTES:

TODAY'S TRAINING

DATE

EXERCISE	SET 1		SET 2		SET 3		SET 4		SET 5		SET 6		SET 7		SET 8	
	WEIGHT		WEIGHT		WEIGHT		WEIGHT		WEIGHT		WEIGHT		WEIGHT		WEIGHT	
	REPS		REPS		REPS		REPS		REPS		REPS		REPS		REPS	

CARDIO/NOTES:

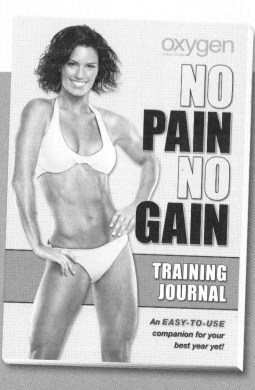

TODAY'S TRAINING

DATE

EXERCISE	SET 1 WEIGHT / REPS	SET 2 WEIGHT / REPS	SET 3 WEIGHT / REPS	SET 4 WEIGHT / REPS	SET 5 WEIGHT / REPS	SET 6 WEIGHT / REPS	SET 7 WEIGHT / REPS	SET 8 WEIGHT / REPS

CARDIO/NOTES:

TODAY'S TRAINING

DATE

EXERCISE	SET 1	SET 2	SET 3	SET 4	SET 5	SET 6	SET 7	SET 8
	WEIGHT	WEIGHT	WEIGHT	WEIGHT	WEIGHT	WEIGHT	WEIGHT	WEIGHT
	REPS	REPS	REPS	REPS	REPS	REPS	REPS	REPS

CARDIO/NOTES:

TODAY'S TRAINING

DATE

EXERCISE	SET 1 WEIGHT REPS	SET 2 WEIGHT REPS	SET 3 WEIGHT REPS	SET 4 WEIGHT REPS	SET 5 WEIGHT REPS	SET 6 WEIGHT REPS	SET 7 WEIGHT REPS	SET 8 WEIGHT REPS

CARDIO/NOTES:

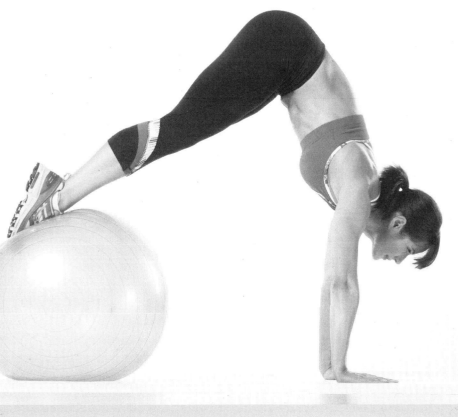

> **If you really want some-thing, you can figure out how to make it happen.**
> — Cher

PHOTOGRAPHY PAUL BUCETA **MODEL** MAGGIE DIUBALDO

TODAY'S TRAINING

EXERCISE	SET 1	SET 2	SET 3	SET 4	SET 5	SET 6	SET 7	SET 8
	WEIGHT	WEIGHT	WEIGHT	WEIGHT	WEIGHT	WEIGHT	WEIGHT	WEIGHT
	REPS	REPS	REPS	REPS	REPS	REPS	REPS	REPS

CARDIO/NOTES:

TODAY'S TRAINING

DATE

EXERCISE	SET 1 WEIGHT	SET 2 WEIGHT	SET 3 WEIGHT	SET 4 WEIGHT	SET 5 WEIGHT	SET 6 WEIGHT	SET 7 WEIGHT	SET 8 WEIGHT
	REPS	REPS	REPS	REPS	REPS	REPS	REPS	REPS

CARDIO/NOTES:

TODAY'S TRAINING

DATE

EXERCISE	SET 1	SET 2	SET 3	SET 4	SET 5	SET 6	SET 7	SET 8
	WEIGHT	WEIGHT	WEIGHT	WEIGHT	WEIGHT	WEIGHT	WEIGHT	WEIGHT
	REPS	REPS	REPS	REPS	REPS	REPS	REPS	REPS

CARDIO/NOTES:

TODAY'S TRAINING

DATE

EXERCISE	SET 1	SET 2	SET 3	SET 4	SET 5	SET 6	SET 7	SET 8
	WEIGHT	WEIGHT	WEIGHT	WEIGHT	WEIGHT	WEIGHT	WEIGHT	WEIGHT
	REPS	REPS	REPS	REPS	REPS	REPS	REPS	REPS

CARDIO/NOTES:

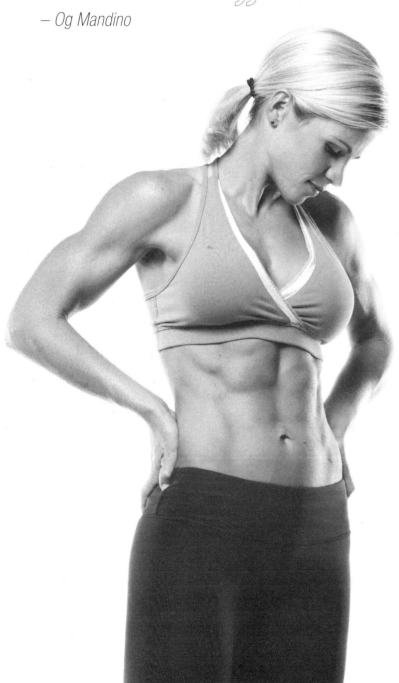

" Failure will never overtake me if my determination to succeed is strong enough. "

– Og Mandino

TODAY'S TRAINING

DATE

EXERCISE	SET 1 WEIGHT REPS	SET 2 WEIGHT REPS	SET 3 WEIGHT REPS	SET 4 WEIGHT REPS	SET 5 WEIGHT REPS	SET 6 WEIGHT REPS	SET 7 WEIGHT REPS	SET 8 WEIGHT REPS

CARDIO/NOTES:

TODAY'S TRAINING

DATE

EXERCISE	SET 1	SET 2	SET 3	SET 4	SET 5	SET 6	SET 7	SET 8
	WEIGHT	WEIGHT	WEIGHT	WEIGHT	WEIGHT	WEIGHT	WEIGHT	WEIGHT
	REPS	REPS	REPS	REPS	REPS	REPS	REPS	REPS

CARDIO/NOTES:

TODAY'S TRAINING

DATE

EXERCISE	SET 1		SET 2		SET 3		SET 4		SET 5		SET 6		SET 7		SET 8	
	WEIGHT	REPS	WEIGHT	REPS	WEIGHT	REPS	WEIGHT	REPS	WEIGHT	REPS	WEIGHT	REPS	WEIGHT	REPS	WEIGHT	REPS

CARDIO/NOTES:

TODAY'S TRAINING

DATE

EXERCISE	SET 1	SET 2	SET 3	SET 4	SET 5	SET 6	SET 7	SET 8
	WEIGHT	WEIGHT	WEIGHT	WEIGHT	WEIGHT	WEIGHT	WEIGHT	WEIGHT
	REPS	REPS	REPS	REPS	REPS	REPS	REPS	REPS

CARDIO/NOTES:

TODAY'S TRAINING

DATE

EXERCISE	SET 1	SET 2	SET 3	SET 4	SET 5	SET 6	SET 7	SET 8
	WEIGHT	WEIGHT	WEIGHT	WEIGHT	WEIGHT	WEIGHT	WEIGHT	WEIGHT
	REPS	REPS	REPS	REPS	REPS	REPS	REPS	REPS

CARDIO/NOTES:

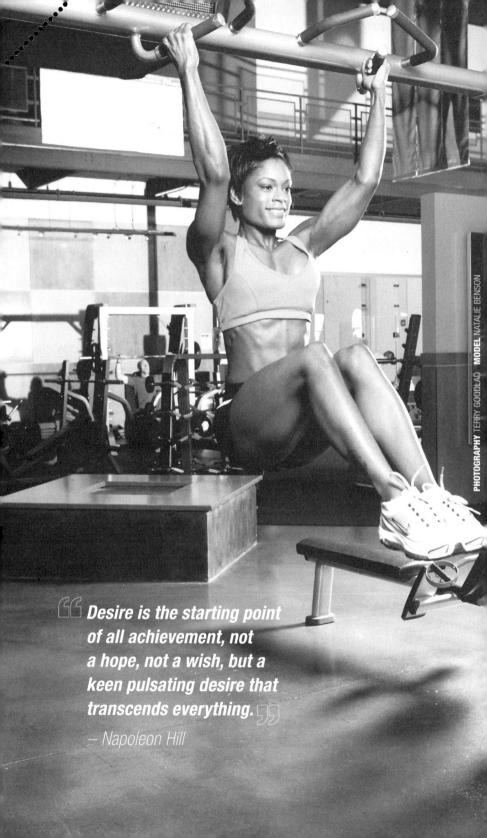

Desire is the starting point of all achievement, not a hope, not a wish, but a keen pulsating desire that transcends everything.

— Napoleon Hill

TODAY'S TRAINING

DATE

EXERCISE	SET 1 WEIGHT / REPS	SET 2 WEIGHT / REPS	SET 3 WEIGHT / REPS	SET 4 WEIGHT / REPS	SET 5 WEIGHT / REPS	SET 6 WEIGHT / REPS	SET 7 WEIGHT / REPS	SET 8 WEIGHT / REPS

CARDIO/NOTES:

TODAY'S TRAINING

DATE

EXERCISE	SET 1 WEIGHT REPS	SET 2 WEIGHT REPS	SET 3 WEIGHT REPS	SET 4 WEIGHT REPS	SET 5 WEIGHT REPS	SET 6 WEIGHT REPS	SET 7 WEIGHT REPS	SET 8 WEIGHT REPS

CARDIO/NOTES:

TODAY'S TRAINING

DATE

EXERCISE	SET 1 WEIGHT REPS	SET 2 WEIGHT REPS	SET 3 WEIGHT REPS	SET 4 WEIGHT REPS	SET 5 WEIGHT REPS	SET 6 WEIGHT REPS	SET 7 WEIGHT REPS	SET 8 WEIGHT REPS

CARDIO/NOTES:

TODAY'S TRAINING

DATE

EXERCISE	SET 1 WEIGHT REPS	SET 2 WEIGHT REPS	SET 3 WEIGHT REPS	SET 4 WEIGHT REPS	SET 5 WEIGHT REPS	SET 6 WEIGHT REPS	SET 7 WEIGHT REPS	SET 8 WEIGHT REPS

CARDIO/NOTES:

TODAY'S TRAINING

DATE

EXERCISE	SET 1 WEIGHT REPS	SET 2 WEIGHT REPS	SET 3 WEIGHT REPS	SET 4 WEIGHT REPS	SET 5 WEIGHT REPS	SET 6 WEIGHT REPS	SET 7 WEIGHT REPS	SET 8 WEIGHT REPS

CARDIO/NOTES:

TODAY'S TRAINING

DATE

EXERCISE	SET 1 WEIGHT	SET 2 WEIGHT	SET 3 WEIGHT	SET 4 WEIGHT	SET 5 WEIGHT	SET 6 WEIGHT	SET 7 WEIGHT	SET 8 WEIGHT
	REPS	REPS	REPS	REPS	REPS	REPS	REPS	REPS

CARDIO/NOTES:

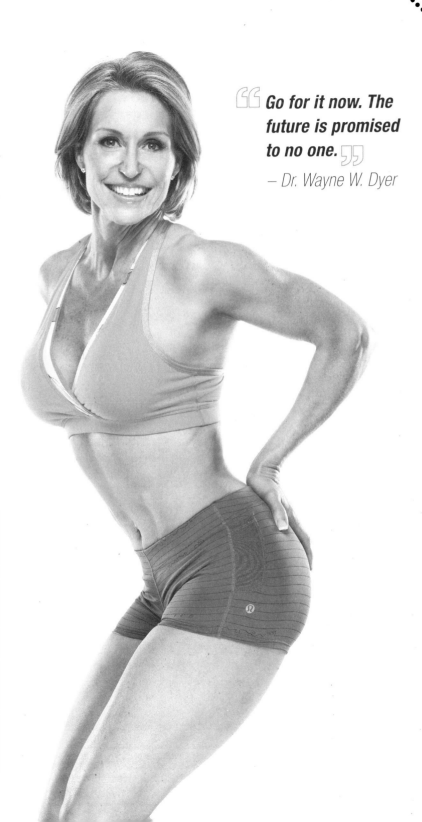

Go for it now. The future is promised to no one.
– Dr. Wayne W. Dyer

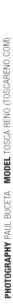

TODAY'S TRAINING

DATE

EXERCISE	SET 1 WEIGHT REPS	SET 2 WEIGHT REPS	SET 3 WEIGHT REPS	SET 4 WEIGHT REPS	SET 5 WEIGHT REPS	SET 6 WEIGHT REPS	SET 7 WEIGHT REPS	SET 8 WEIGHT REPS

CARDIO/NOTES:

TODAY'S TRAINING

DATE

EXERCISE	SET 1 WEIGHT	SET 2 WEIGHT	SET 3 WEIGHT	SET 4 WEIGHT	SET 5 WEIGHT	SET 6 WEIGHT	SET 7 WEIGHT	SET 8 WEIGHT
	REPS	REPS	REPS	REPS	REPS	REPS	REPS	REPS

CARDIO/NOTES:

TODAY'S TRAINING

DATE

EXERCISE	SET 1 WEIGHT REPS	SET 2 WEIGHT REPS	SET 3 WEIGHT REPS	SET 4 WEIGHT REPS	SET 5 WEIGHT REPS	SET 6 WEIGHT REPS	SET 7 WEIGHT REPS	SET 8 WEIGHT REPS

CARDIO/NOTES:

TODAY'S TRAINING

DATE

EXERCISE	SET 1		SET 2		SET 3		SET 4		SET 5		SET 6		SET 7		SET 8	
	WEIGHT	REPS	WEIGHT	REPS	WEIGHT	REPS	WEIGHT	REPS	WEIGHT	REPS	WEIGHT	REPS	WEIGHT	REPS	WEIGHT	REPS

CARDIO/NOTES:

TODAY'S TRAINING

DATE

EXERCISE	SET 1 WEIGHT REPS	SET 2 WEIGHT REPS	SET 3 WEIGHT REPS	SET 4 WEIGHT REPS	SET 5 WEIGHT REPS	SET 6 WEIGHT REPS	SET 7 WEIGHT REPS	SET 8 WEIGHT REPS

CARDIO/NOTES:

TODAY'S TRAINING

DATE

EXERCISE	SET 1 WEIGHT	SET 2 WEIGHT	SET 3 WEIGHT	SET 4 WEIGHT	SET 5 WEIGHT	SET 6 WEIGHT	SET 7 WEIGHT	SET 8 WEIGHT
	REPS	REPS	REPS	REPS	REPS	REPS	REPS	REPS

CARDIO/NOTES:

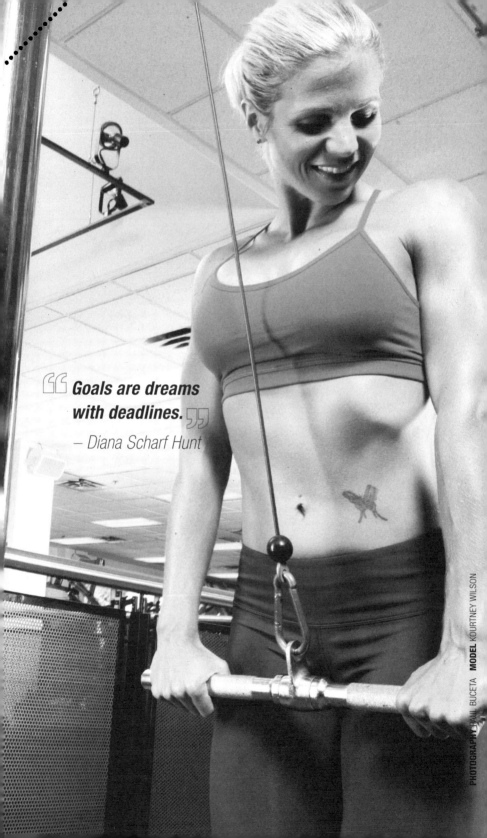

> **Goals are dreams with deadlines.**
> – Diana Scharf Hunt

TODAY'S TRAINING

DATE

EXERCISE	SET 1	SET 2	SET 3	SET 4	SET 5	SET 6	SET 7	SET 8
	WEIGHT	WEIGHT	WEIGHT	WEIGHT	WEIGHT	WEIGHT	WEIGHT	WEIGHT
	REPS	REPS	REPS	REPS	REPS	REPS	REPS	REPS

CARDIO/NOTES:

TODAY'S TRAINING

DATE

EXERCISE	SET 1	SET 2	SET 3	SET 4	SET 5	SET 6	SET 7	SET 8
	WEIGHT	WEIGHT	WEIGHT	WEIGHT	WEIGHT	WEIGHT	WEIGHT	WEIGHT
	REPS	REPS	REPS	REPS	REPS	REPS	REPS	REPS

CARDIO/NOTES:

TODAY'S TRAINING

DATE

EXERCISE	SET 1	SET 2	SET 3	SET 4	SET 5	SET 6	SET 7	SET 8
	WEIGHT	WEIGHT	WEIGHT	WEIGHT	WEIGHT	WEIGHT	WEIGHT	WEIGHT
	REPS	REPS	REPS	REPS	REPS	REPS	REPS	REPS

CARDIO/NOTES:

TODAY'S TRAINING

DATE

EXERCISE	SET 1	SET 2	SET 3	SET 4	SET 5	SET 6	SET 7	SET 8
	WEIGHT	WEIGHT	WEIGHT	WEIGHT	WEIGHT	WEIGHT	WEIGHT	WEIGHT
	REPS	REPS	REPS	REPS	REPS	REPS	REPS	REPS

CARDIO/NOTES:

TODAY'S TRAINING

DATE

EXERCISE	SET 1	SET 2	SET 3	SET 4	SET 5	SET 6	SET 7	SET 8
	WEIGHT	WEIGHT	WEIGHT	WEIGHT	WEIGHT	WEIGHT	WEIGHT	WEIGHT
	REPS	REPS	REPS	REPS	REPS	REPS	REPS	REPS

CARDIO/NOTES:

TODAY'S TRAINING

EXERCISE	SET 1	SET 2	SET 3	SET 4	SET 5	SET 6	SET 7	SET 8
	WEIGHT	WEIGHT	WEIGHT	WEIGHT	WEIGHT	WEIGHT	WEIGHT	WEIGHT
	REPS	REPS	REPS	REPS	REPS	REPS	REPS	REPS

CARDIO/NOTES:

Difficulties are meant to rouse, not discourage. The human spirit is to grow strong by conflict.

– William E. Channing

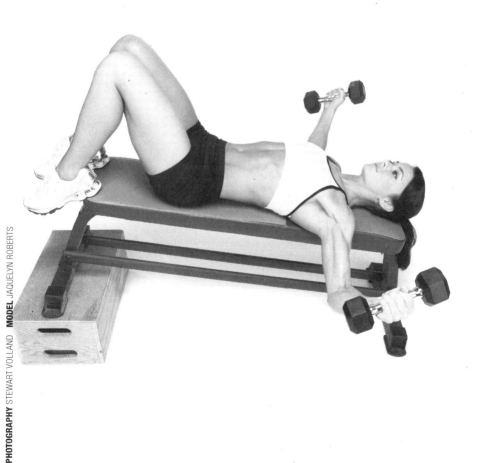

TODAY'S TRAINING

DATE

EXERCISE	SET 1		SET 2		SET 3		SET 4		SET 5		SET 6		SET 7		SET 8	
	WEIGHT	REPS	WEIGHT	REPS	WEIGHT	REPS	WEIGHT	REPS	WEIGHT	REPS	WEIGHT	REPS	WEIGHT	REPS	WEIGHT	REPS

CARDIO/NOTES:

TODAY'S TRAINING

DATE

EXERCISE	SET 1 WEIGHT REPS	SET 2 WEIGHT REPS	SET 3 WEIGHT REPS	SET 4 WEIGHT REPS	SET 5 WEIGHT REPS	SET 6 WEIGHT REPS	SET 7 WEIGHT REPS	SET 8 WEIGHT REPS

CARDIO/NOTES:

TODAY'S TRAINING

DATE

EXERCISE	SET 1	SET 2	SET 3	SET 4	SET 5	SET 6	SET 7	SET 8
	WEIGHT	WEIGHT	WEIGHT	WEIGHT	WEIGHT	WEIGHT	WEIGHT	WEIGHT
	REPS	REPS	REPS	REPS	REPS	REPS	REPS	REPS

CARDIO/NOTES:

TODAY'S TRAINING

DATE

EXERCISE	SET 1	SET 2	SET 3	SET 4	SET 5	SET 6	SET 7	SET 8
	WEIGHT	WEIGHT	WEIGHT	WEIGHT	WEIGHT	WEIGHT	WEIGHT	WEIGHT
	REPS	REPS	REPS	REPS	REPS	REPS	REPS	REPS

CARDIO/NOTES:

TODAY'S TRAINING

EXERCISE	SET 1 WEIGHT REPS	SET 2 WEIGHT REPS	SET 3 WEIGHT REPS	SET 4 WEIGHT REPS	SET 5 WEIGHT REPS	SET 6 WEIGHT REPS	SET 7 WEIGHT REPS	SET 8 WEIGHT REPS

CARDIO/NOTES:

TODAY'S TRAINING

DATE

EXERCISE	SET 1	SET 2	SET 3	SET 4	SET 5	SET 6	SET 7	SET 8
	WEIGHT	WEIGHT	WEIGHT	WEIGHT	WEIGHT	WEIGHT	WEIGHT	WEIGHT
	REPS	REPS	REPS	REPS	REPS	REPS	REPS	REPS

CARDIO/NOTES:

TODAY'S TRAINING

DATE

EXERCISE	SET 1	SET 2	SET 3	SET 4	SET 5	SET 6	SET 7	SET 8
	WEIGHT	WEIGHT	WEIGHT	WEIGHT	WEIGHT	WEIGHT	WEIGHT	WEIGHT
	REPS	REPS	REPS	REPS	REPS	REPS	REPS	REPS

CARDIO/NOTES:

TODAY'S TRAINING

DATE

EXERCISE	SET 1		SET 2		SET 3		SET 4		SET 5		SET 6		SET 7		SET 8	
	WEIGHT	REPS	WEIGHT	REPS	WEIGHT	REPS	WEIGHT	REPS	WEIGHT	REPS	WEIGHT	REPS	WEIGHT	REPS	WEIGHT	REPS

CARDIO/NOTES:

CALORIES BURNED

EXERCISE	DURATION & CALORIES BURNED		
	30 MINUTES	45 MINUTES	60 MINUTES
Calisthenics (light)	120 calories	180 calories	240 calories
Cycling (5 mph)	120 calories	180 calories	240 calories
Cycling (8-8.5 mph)	180 calories	270 calories	360 calories
Cycling (12 mph)	300 calories	450 calories	600 calories
Cycling (14 mph)	360 calories	540 calories	720 calories
Cycling (16 mph)	450 calories	675 calories	900 calories
Dancing (light)	150 calories	225 calories	300 calories
Dancing (moderate-heavy)	240 calories	360 calories	480 calories
Hiking	210 calories	315 calories	420 calories
Jogging (5 mph)	300 calories	450 calories	600 calories
Rollerblading (light)	180 calories	270 calories	360 calories
Rollerblading (heavy)	330 calories	495 calories	660 calories
Running (5.5 mph)	330 calories	495 calories	660 calories
Running (6 mph)	390 calories	585 calories	780 calories
Running (7 mph)	450 calories	675 calories	900 calories
Running (8 mph)	480 calories	720 calories	960 calories
Running (9 mph)	510 calories	765 calories	1020 calories
Running (10 mph)	540 calories	810 calories	1080 calories
Stair climbing (light)	180 calories	270 calories	360 calories
Stair climing (moderate)	240 calories	360 calories	480 calories
Stair climbing (heavy)	300 calories	450 calories	600 calories
Swimming (light)	180 calories	270 calories	360 calories
Walking (1-2 mph)	90 calories	135 calories	180 calories
Walking (2-3 mph)	120 calories	180 calories	240 calories
Walking (3.5-4 mph)	180 calories	270 calories	360 calories
Walking (4-4.5 mph)	210 calories	315 calories	420 calories
Walking (5 mph)	240 calories	360 calories	480 calories

NOTES

NOTES

NOTES